Reflections

on

Mary's Help Hospital

and

Seton Medical Center

To Toni & Dan Foster,

Sharing memories

Marie Mahoney.

Oct. 1994

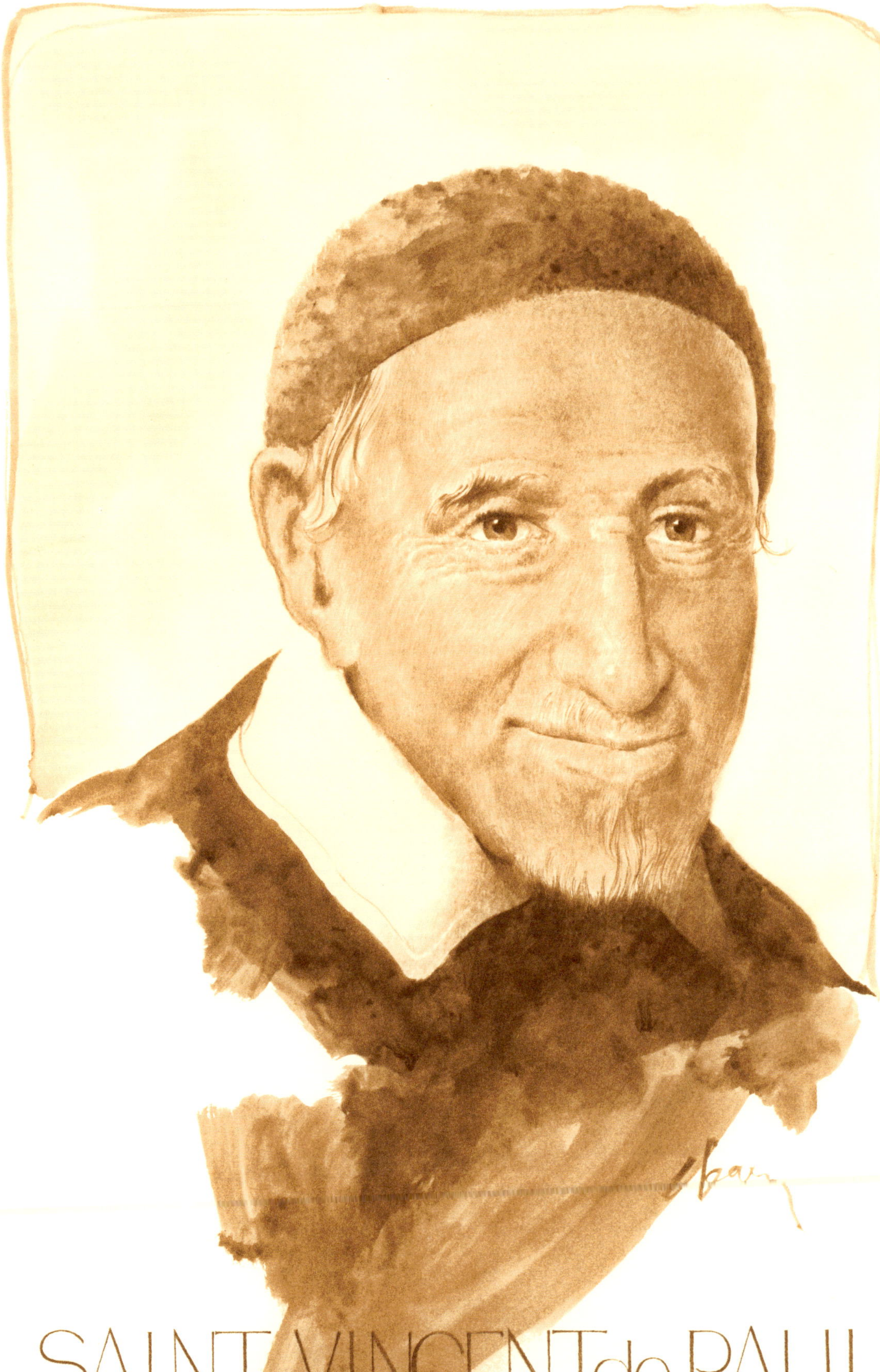

SAINT VINCENT de PAUL

Reflections on Mary's Help Hospital and Seton Medical Center 1893–1985

by

Marie M. Mahoney

SETON MEDICAL CENTER
Daly City, California
Sponsored and Operated by the Daughters of Charity of Saint Vincent de Paul

Library of Congress Cataloging in Publication Data

Mahoney, Marie M.
Reflections on Mary's Help Hospital and
Seton Medical Center,
1893-1985.

Bibliography: p 168
1. Mary's Help Hospital (Daly City, Calif.)—History.
2. Seton Medical Center—History. I. Title.
[DNLM: 1. Mary's Help Hospital (Daly City, Calif.)
2. Seton Medical Center. 3. Hospitals—history—
California. WX 28 AC2 M393r]
RA982.D25M375 1985 362.1'1'0979469 86-8256
ISBN 0-9616516-0-1

Editorial Supervision for Seton Medical Center
Claire Robbat

Cover Design
Concept from the Formation group of the Daughters of Charity
Executed by Madeleine Corson

Frontispiece
St. Vincent de Paul, Founder of the Daughters of Charity
Portrait by Joseph S. Cleary

Dedication

This account is dedicated to:
The Daughters of Charity who served at
Mary's Help Hospital
in San Francisco
and who were and are assigned to
Seton Medical Center
in Daly City.
All my co-workers
and others whose lives were touched by
Mary's Help Hospital
&
Seton Medical Center.
All those who shared their memories
to help create this account of
Mary's Help Hospital
&
Seton Medical Center.

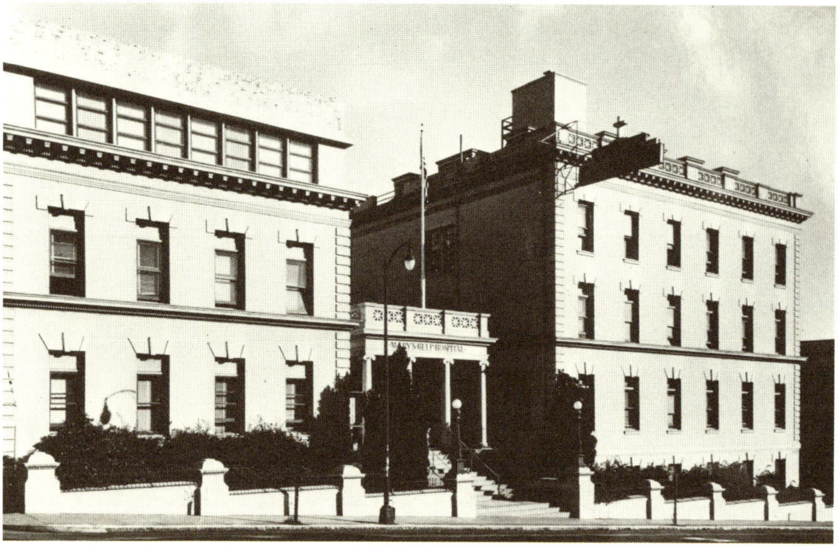

Mary's Help Hospital
San Francisco

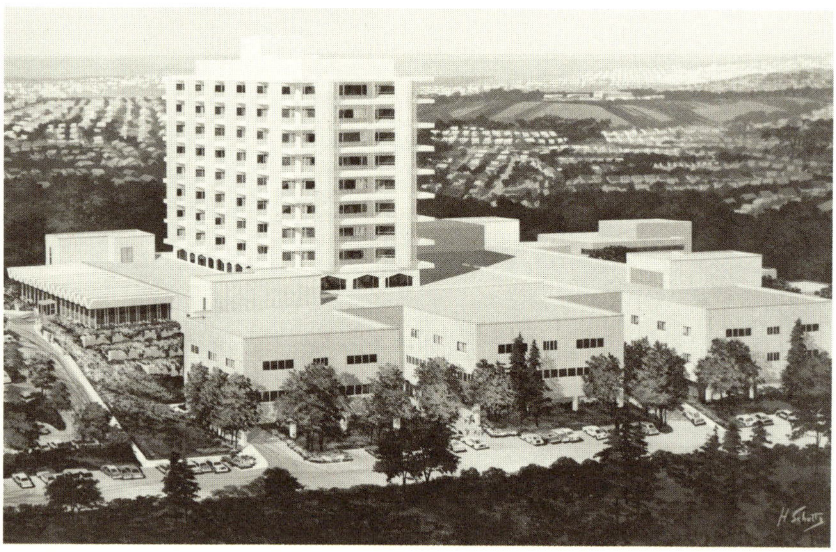

Seton Medical Center
Daly City

Foreword

History is especially fascinating when it springs from the sharing of memories by one who has lived it. No one is more qualified to write the story of Mary's Help Hospital and Seton Medical Center than Marie Mahoney. In 1986 she will celebrate 50 years of loving service to the hospital. She has not only lived this story—she was a participant in its creation.

Marie's formal association with the hospital began when she entered the Mary's Help Hospital School of Nursing. After graduation and while working as an emergency room nurse, she attended workers who had been injured in the building of the Golden Gate and Bay Bridges. In addition to her work as a nurse, Marie continued with further education and earned a master's degree in education.

As an instructor in the Mary's Help Hospital School of Nursing, Marie influenced an entire generation of Bay Area nurses. From her they learned the importance of maintaining high standards of care. Her concern for the needs of each patient was—and is—a living example of the motto of the Daughters: *The Charity of Christ Urges Us.*

While she was Director of Education, Marie played a major part in the organization of the hospital's move from San Francisco to Daly City in 1965. In the years that followed, she has been a driving force in the effort to ensure that the values of St. Vincent de Paul, founder of the Daughters of Charity, permeate every facet of the hospital's environment.

Since 1982 Marie has served as Assistant Administrator and then as Associate Administrator at the newly named Seton Medical Center. She is currently Assistant to the President of Mission Services Corporation, the parent organization, which includes Seton Medical Center, St. Catherine Hospital On Half Moon Bay, the San Francisco Heart Institute, the Western Hansen's Disease Institute, and several other subsidiaries.

In this volume Marie offers us the gift of a personally witnessed account of the growth of a small hospital in San Francisco to what is today a leading medical center, located in Daly City and serving patients from all over the world.

Marie Mahoney has been there all along—dedicated to the mission of the Daughters of Charity: to bring hope and loving care to those in need. Her telling the story of the past half century should be an inspiration to those who will carry on the mission of Seton Medical Center in the years to come.

Sister Marilynn Emminger, D.C.
Health Councillor, Province of the West
Daughters of Charity of Saint Vincent de Paul

Los Altos Hills, California
December 1985

Preface

This chronicle represents a challenge and a unique opportunity for me. To be requested to write a history of Mary's Help Hospital, now Seton Medical Center, where I have spent my life, permits me to record the events that shaped the growth of an outstanding institution—one which has developed from a small hospital into a major medical center, but one that has always been characterized by our spirit of caring.

I believe history to be "the most human of sciences," not only because it touches social acts but because it keeps in touch with the people and all their activities. This simple account does attempt to chronicle some of the events and, more significantly, the people who make up our story.

My major concern is that I shall be unable to include all the events and all the people who have made their contributions: the Daughters of Charity, the physicians, the Boards of Trustees, the employees, the volunteers, and all the others who have given so much.

In anticipation of my failing to mention that which should be recorded, I am including as a disclaimer the words of Thomas Hardy:

> *Much is there waits you that we have missed,*
> *Much lore we leave you worth the knowing,*
> *Much, much has lain outside our ken.*
>
> —AN ANCIENT TO ANCIENTS

Marie M. Mahoney

Daly City, California
December 1985

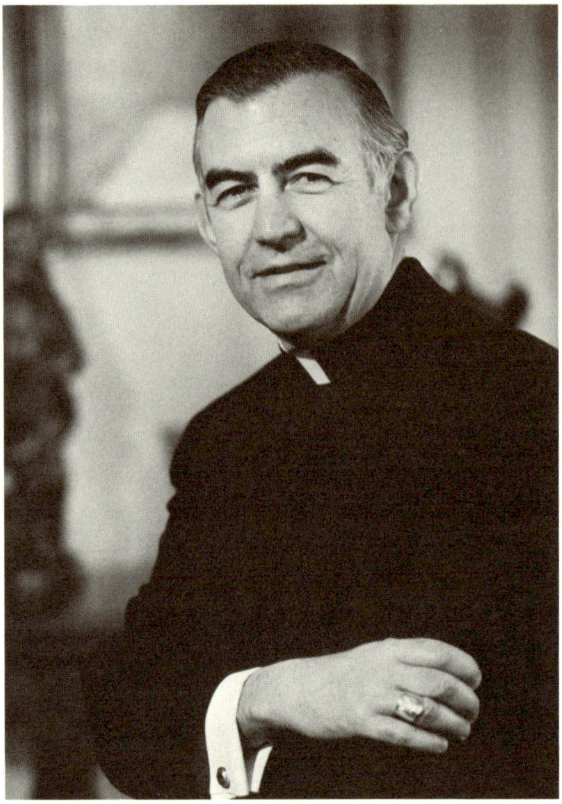

MOST REVEREND JOHN R. QUINN, D.D.
Archbishop of San Francisco

Table of Contents

I

Our Origin: Troubled Times 1893–1912

MARY'S HELP HOSPITAL was one of several legacies given by Mrs. Kate Johnson to the Archdiocese of San Francisco. In 1862, Robert G. Johnson married Miss Catherine (Kate) Birdsell. Johnson's father was consul for Norway and Sweden, an importer of iron and steel, and the owner of the George Johnson Saddlery and Harness business of San Francisco. Robert Johnson, like his father, became a successful businessman and acquired several large real estate properties in San Francisco. Kate, later widowed from Robert Johnson, was the benefactress who provided the finances and the plan for the first Mary's Help Hospital. In 1889, she bequeathed to Archbishop Patrick William Riordan funds to be held in trust by him for the purpose of establishing Mary's Help Hospital. Kate Johnson was a convert to Catholicism and from the time of her husband's death, she was a major donor to the Catholic Church in California.

The plan Mrs. Johnson offered to Archbishop Riordan was that she would provide the property and endow a "sunlight" hospital for women and children in San Francisco. The first site she selected, on Castro Street, was not accepted by Archbishop Riordan. She subsequently offered the Guerrero Street property between 13th and 14th Streets, and the Archbishop agreed.

Plans for the hospital building moved slowly. Mrs. Johnson died on December 3, 1893, prior to the first meeting of the Board of Directors, which had been appointed by Archbishop Riordan to manage the project. The will of Mrs. Johnson, dated July 19, 1892, stated:

> *. . . money and property is to be trusted, paid, conveyed and delivered over to a corporation to be hereafter formed by a society to be composed of the Roman Catholic Archbishop of San Francisco and Mr. Robert C. Tobin, Dr. C. F. Buckley, Dr. W. S. Thorne and Dr. Luke Robinson or the survivors of them and such other*

> *persons as they or their survivors and successors in their discretion shall elect to fill the vacancies in said society, said corporation to be formed under the laws of the State of California, the name of such corporation to be Mary's Help Hospital; the purpose for which said corporation shall be formed is to receive endowments and acquire property for and establish, erect, maintain and conduct a free hospital for all sick women and children of the poor, without regard to religion, nationality or color, excepting such as the officers of the hospital consider dangerous to other inmates; such hospital to be conducted by the Roman Catholic Sisters of St. Vincent de Paul, commonly called the Sisters of Charity, under the direction of the Board of Directors of said corporation. . . .*

The Articles of Incorporation for Mary's Help Hospital were signed by Archbishop Riordan and Mr. Robert Tobin on December 28, 1893, at 1100 Franklin Street in San Francisco.

There were two stipulations for the endowment. First, the hospital would be built in the "sunshine area" of the Mission District of San Francisco, and designed in the form of a St. Andrew's Cross to ensure maximum sunlight in every room. Second, the Archbishop would ask the Daughters of Charity of St. Vincent de Paul, whose work with the sick and poor Mrs. Johnson had observed throughout Europe, to manage the hospital.

Mrs. Johnson's condition that the hospital be a "sunlight" one no doubt stemmed from her observations of the use of sunlight as therapy which she saw practiced during her numerous European journeys. In this period, exposure to sunlight was regarded as a powerful curative agent. She was also aware that the poor living in the slums of European cities were deprived of sunlight.

The building was to be constructed in the form of a St. Andrew's Cross, with a center core, a rotunda, and projecting wings of rooms. This plan provided each room and each ward bed with a window and maximum sunlight.

The order of the Daughters of Charity was founded in Paris, France on November 29, 1633. The Daughters were a small group of "good village girls" directed by St. Vincent de Paul and formed by St. Louise de Marillac to serve the spiritual and corporal needs of the poor and the

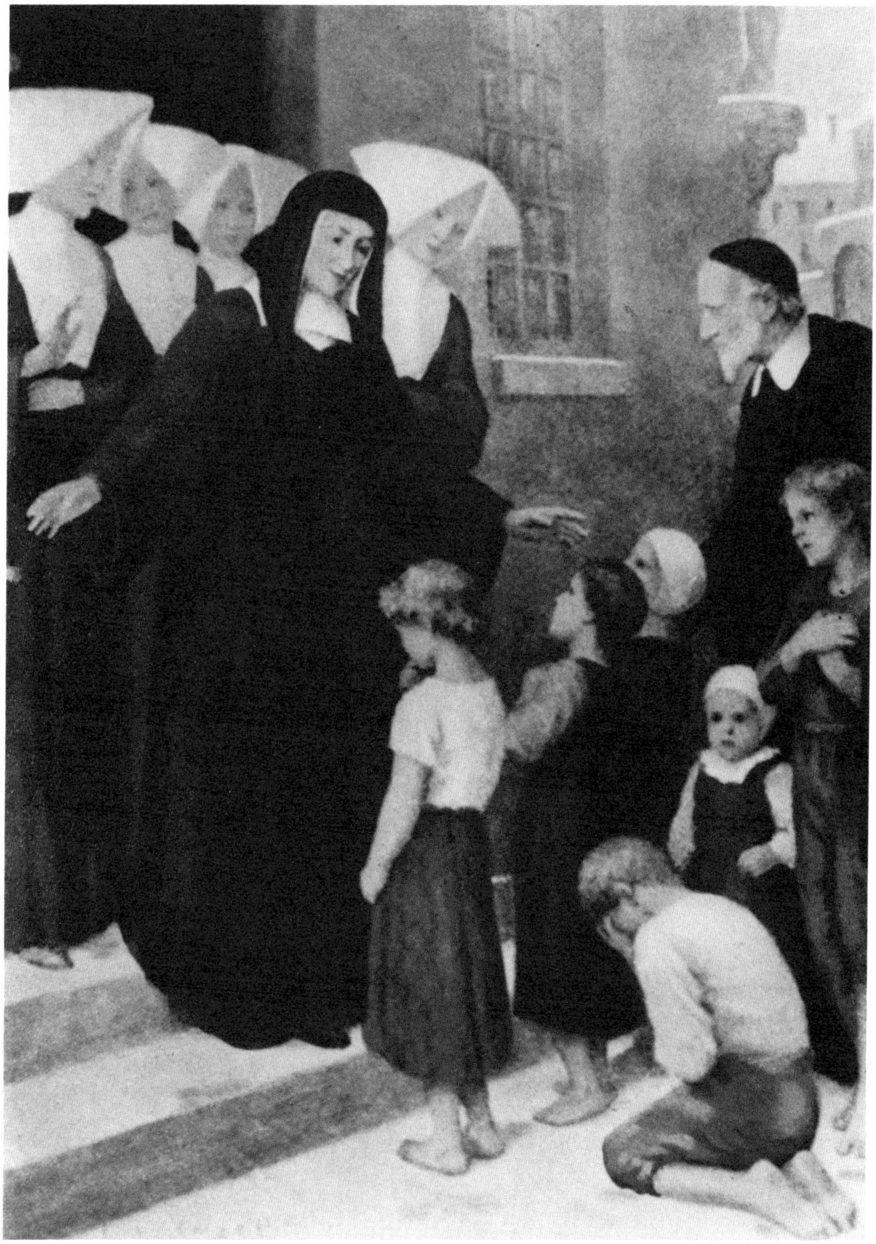

St. Vincent de Paul bringing orphans to St. Louise de Marillac
and the Daughters of Charity in France.

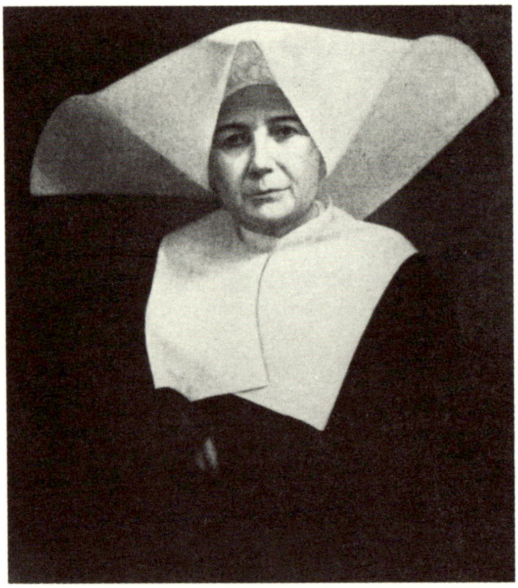

SISTER FRANCIS McENNIS
Leader of the first group of Sisters to arrive in San Francisco, August 18, 1852.

sick. It was St. Vincent's plan that the Daughters of Charity would break away from the traditional cloistered life of religious orders of women in the church. The Daughters were to work where the people needed them most—in their homes, their villages, their schools, and their hospitals. St. Vincent de Paul counseled:

> *You will have for chapel, the parish church; for cloister, streets of the city and wards of the hospital; for cell, a rented room; for grate, the fear of God; for veil, holy modesty; for grille, holy obedience.*

The Daughters of Charity came to San Francisco in 1852 from Emmitsburg, Maryland, at the request of Archbishop Joseph Sadoc Alemany O.P., first Archbishop of San Francisco. Travel from Maryland to California in 1852 was difficult for the first seven Daughters of Charity. The long trip required sailing to Panama, traveling across the Isthmus on foot and donkey to the Pacific, and then sailing to San Francisco. Sister Ignatia and Sister Honorine died of cholera on the journey. On August 18, 1852, the five remaining Daughters—Sisters Francis McEnnis, Fidelis Buckley, Sebastian Doyle, Bernice Williams, and Corsina McDay—reached San Francisco. Father Maginnis, the Pastor of Saint Patrick's Church, welcomed them to their first house in San Francisco. It was a dilapitated little frame building at Market and Montgomery Streets (the site of the present Sheraton Palace Hotel). Fifteen orphan girls were waiting along with Father Maginnis for the Sisters. The work of the social ministry of the Daughters of Charity in San Francisco began in 1852, on the day they arrived.

On October 7, 1852, the Daughters opened a day school in their small structure. Father Maginnis and an Irish schoolmaster, Mr. Barry, taught the boys, and the Sisters taught the girls. At the end of the first term there were ninety students.

On March 17, 1855, the second group of Daughters arrived—Sister Frederica, Sister Philita, Sister Mary Angela, Sister Vincent, and Sister Mary Joseph. They traveled on the first train to cross the Isthmus of Panama. The education of the boys was then transferred to

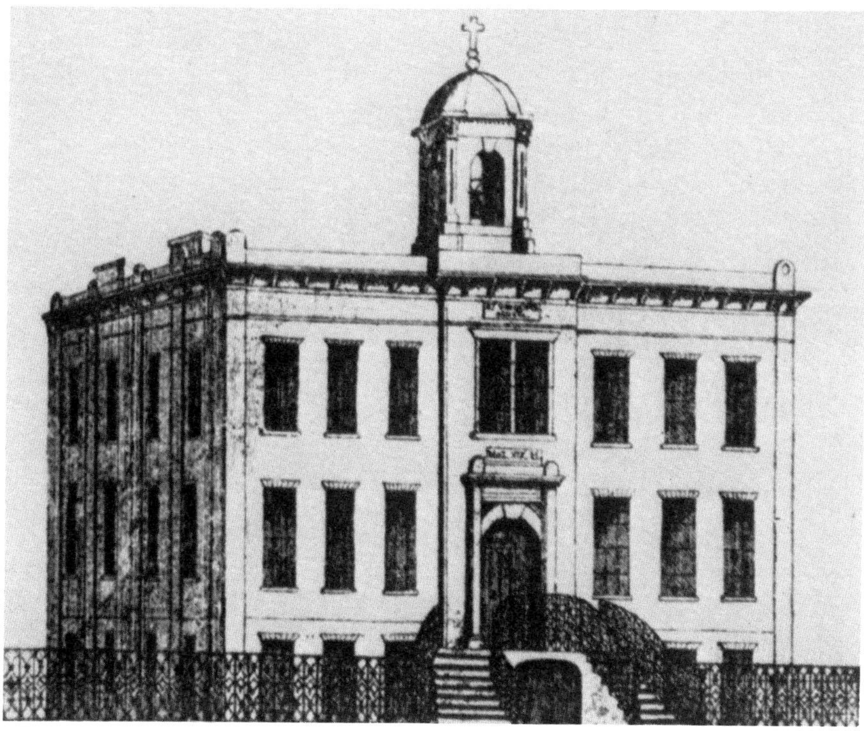

The first Daughters of Charity school and orphanage in San Francisco, located on the present site of the Sheraton Palace Hotel, Market and Montgomery Streets.

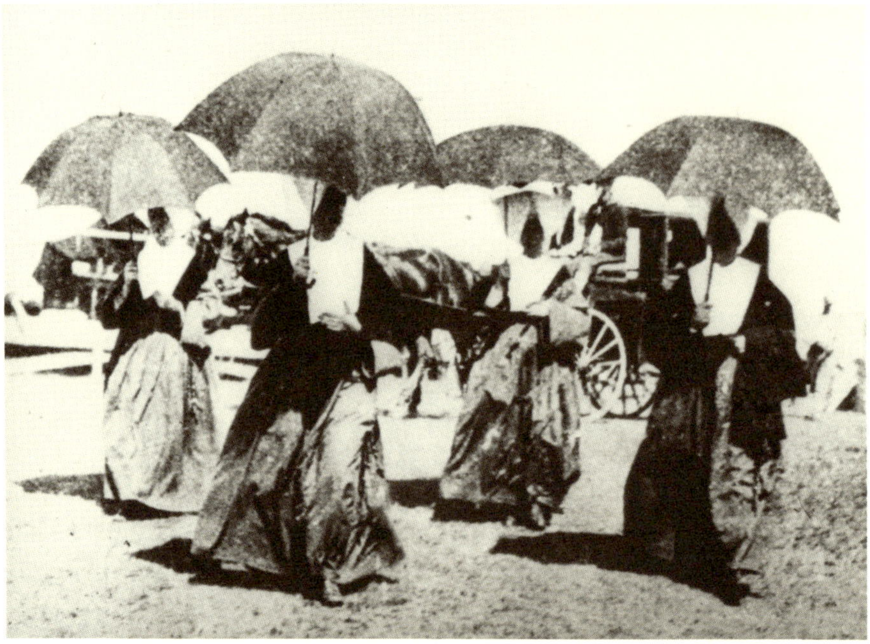

Daughters of Charity: Early days in San Francisco.

the Sisters. The need for a larger school became critical. When a collection was taken up for this purpose at St. Francis Church on Vallejo Street in San Francisco, Archbishop Alemany removed his gold pectoral cross and chain, donating them as his contribution. In 1858, the school building on Jessie Street opened with an enrollment of seventy-five orphans and three hundred day-school students.

In 1899, Archbishop Riordan, second Archbishop of San Francisco, contacted Sister Mariana Flynn, Visitatrix of the Daughters of Charity at the provincial house in Emmitsburg, Maryland, to request that she send Sisters to staff and manage the hospital endowed by Mrs. Johnson. Originally, there was one province of the Daughters of Charity in the United States, with the provincial house located in Emmitsburg, Maryland. Due to the westward expansion of the United States and the accompanying growth of the work of the Daughters of Charity, a second province was formed on July 3, 1910. The country was then divided into two provinces: the Eastern Province with the provincial house at St. Joseph's Central House in Emmitsburg,

Maryland, and the Western Province with the provincial house at Marillac Seminary, Normandy, situated near St. Louis, Missouri. Sister Mariana traveled to California to confer with the Archbishop in 1901. She became ill in Los Angeles, and Archbishop Riordan visited her there. Before her death she agreed that the Daughters of Charity would accept the management of Mary's Help Hospital.

In addition to the money to purchase the land and build the hospital, Mrs. Johnson also donated a number of income properties to produce on-going revenue to finance the project.

It is also worth noting that shortly before her death Mrs. Johnson made another bequest to Archbishop Riordan, a tract of land in Menlo Park, thirty miles south of San Francisco. Shortly thereafter, St. Patrick's Seminary was built on this property. It continues to be the major seminary for the education of priests in this Archdiocese.

The first meeting of the Board of Mary's Help Hospital Corporation took place in the Spring of 1894, six months after the death of Mrs. Johnson. The five-member Board was chaired by Archbishop Patrick Riordan and Robert Tobin, of the Hibernia Bank Tobins, who was appointed Secretary and empowered to act in the absence of the Archbishop. In 1900, Mr. Tobin was replaced as Secretary of the Board by Father Patrick Mulligan.

Nine years elapsed between the first meeting of the Board of the Corporation and the 1903 laying of the hospital cornerstone on Guerrero Street between Duboce Avenue (formerly called 13th Street) and 14th Street. Construction began; Mr. Charles J. I. Devlin was the architect. The hospital was ready to be opened in the Spring of 1906.

The events of April 18, 1906—the earthquake and fire—destroyed the almost-completed hospital. Three of the four other missions of the Daughters of Charity in San Francisco were not destroyed. These included the Roman Catholic Orphan Asylum, Mount St. Joseph's Infant Asylum, and St. Francis Technical School. The fourth structure—St. Vincent's School at 671 Mission Street—was demolished by the earthquake.

This description of San Francisco on April 19, 1906, was sent to the French newspaper, *Figaro*, by Messrs. H. and G. Roulleaux-Dugage. They were the two sons of the Deputy of Orne and were returning from Japan on board the vessel *China*. Being unable to go ashore for two days, they observed the scene from the harbor. Their description was included in the report of events that was sent to the Motherhouse on Rue de Bac in Paris:

> . . . *With the pilot came the appalling news: Since yesterday morning, San Francisco is in flames—a violent earthquake suddenly aroused the sleeping city, and for forty-five seconds, an eternity—shook the ground to its upheaval, split the walls, and as if they had been castles made of pasteboard, demolished the stateliest edifices, crushing hundreds beneath the ruins, and, on the same instant, fire bursts forth: for twenty-four hours it holds sway. All the hotels, the banks and all the public buildings are destroyed, all material aid cut off, entire sections consumed; one-half the population without shelter; without provisions; Chinatown is but a heap of ruins, the dead may be reckoned by thousands. Means of communication no longer exist; the railroads have been destroyed by the quake, the cables are broken, the docks have fallen in, and no boats can land. Martial law is proclaimed; over one hundred lawless thieves and instigators of disorder have been shot in the streets . . . and the fire is gaining ground—no one thinks of going ashore.*
>
> *Everyone is in consternation, but American coolness checks the anguish of those who have relatives, or children in the burning city, and silence—a silence more impressive than cries and tears—greets the fearful tidings. . . . The smoke becomes more dense. As we enter the Golden Gate, the whole panorama of San Francisco is unfolded to our view. Only the shore is distinctly visible; clouds, yellow, violet, and grey, whirl around until they blend with a soiled blue coloring that covered a large space, and in this coloring, a long black trail, like a smoking lampwick, ascends from an oil manufacturer. In the near perspective, upon a tower still standing, the large clock stopped at the fatal hour (5h. 16. a.m.). Beyond this, the Palace Hotel appears but an iron skeleton surmounted by a black dome, a large hotel overlooking the scene, and of which only the stone framework is left, presents a vague phantom appearance, like a triumphal arch—a triumphal arch to commemorate the destruction wrought by death!*

The whole center of the city is one burning furnace and the flames are as visible as though it were midnight. One church remains intact; we see it smoke a long time seeming to hesitate, then, suddenly, the large gothic clock ignites from rim to rim, the moellons are displaced, one moment more and the whole edifice gives way. Houses crumble down like funeral pyres consumed. Over a distance of several kilometers, there is before us but one immense brazier, and the sun, which shines above merged into a halo of smoke, burns with a deeper yellowish flame and floods us with his reflex of the conflagration. The China *itself seems to be on fire and one experiences an acrid stifling sensation in the throat. The fog horns send forth a sinister yell, now low, now sharp and shrill, like dogs wounded to the death. With the sound of cannon, comes a continuous thundering forth of explosions, from powder magazines; gas conduits burst, and dynamite destroys entire streets, striving by these gaps to stay the progress of the fire. Crowded ferry-boats and barques almost sinking pass near us, and those who have been so favored as to be able to leave the city cry out pell-mell the details of the horrible tragedy. Three hundred thousand people camp in the parks and public squares; unable to flee further, they await some unexpected assistance; the hospitals which had sheltered the aged and little children have been destroyed and many of the sick, so hastily transported, died on the way; others who believed themselves safe were burned in their improvised refuges; charred bodies block up the streets, and amid the frenzied disorder of the hour scenes of horror are enacted; in their eagerness to possess themselves of rings and jewels, wretches were seen cutting off the fingers of dead women, or even of those who had only swooned away; stores were pillaged, and looters, caught in the act, were shot down without any form of trial. As if guided by a train of powder the flames advance; an irresistible power seems constantly to create new hearthstones.*

And the setting sun seems to mingle its farewell gleams with the blazing conflagration; the smoke every instant becoming more dense ascends until lost in the clouds. The sea is a liquid fire. Night comes on bringing with it the apotheosis of nightmare—a vision, horrific and grandiose like Thurner's dream. The live coals seem of a more

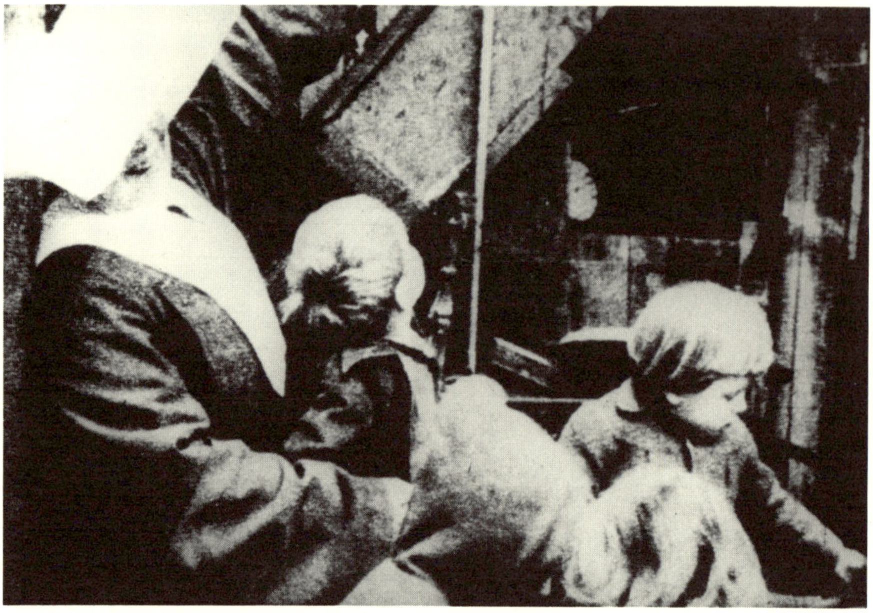

The Daughters of Charity work where people need them most.

dazzling red, and amid the darkness the furnace burns with a vigorous intensity.

The church bells still uninjured sound the alarm while onward rush the flames. Heartrending as agonizing cries, the shrieks of the boat-whistles grow still more gloomy. Portions of blackened wood and cinders float over the water. What anguish for us, powerless spectators, whilst the mind pictures what is going on around us; sublime devotedness and scenes of wild unrest—the angel and the beast awaking in the presence of death.

In old Brahminical India funeral pyres are daily consumed along the banks of the sacred Ganges, but this is the humanity of days gone-by, the isolation of the individual as he makes his lonely departure. Here it is modern life—life in its very excess, wherein all efforts are concentrated in the struggle for existence: this is the life which is absorbed in the frightful brazier we are contemplating. It is the agony of Titan in a city of the twentieth century.

Many of the earthquake victims had to be transported out of the city to San Mateo and San Jose for care. The Daughters of Charity volunteered their services and were able to commandeer a "rag wagon" for five dollars to transport themselves to the injured.

The fact that the Daughters of Charity were able to obtain transportation at this time was no small accomplishment. A major problem in San Francisco after the earthquake was the absence of any form of transportation. Survivors were willing to pay any price for a wagon, a wheelbarrow, or any conveyance with wheels or casters to move their remaining possessions. The ability of the Daughters of Charity to have had their "rag wagon" at this time in San Francisco's history is to be remembered.

Mrs. Johnson's operational plans for Mary's Help Hospital, along with the physical plant itself, were destroyed by the earthquake and fire. The destruction of the original building required that a new structure be refinanced and the original plan restructured. The fire also destroyed many of the income-producing properties Mrs. Johnson had bequeathed to support the hospital. Not only was there a decrease in revenue for Mary's Help Hospital, but tax liabilities as well. New financing had to be obtained.

There were long and complicated court proceedings following the earthquake. Litigation revolved around the problem of the Board's right to use the endowment to build a hospital that would differ from the type specified in Mrs. Johnson's will. The court finally agreed to the petitions of the Corporation that the hospital would be rebuilt. The totally free hospital for women and children that Kate Johnson had envisioned became a "part-pay" general hospital. However, the court would not relent on the physical plan of the hospital and stipulated that the St. Andrew's Cross design be maintained. While the plan of a central rotunda and projecting wings of rooms ensured maximum sunlight, this was a very limiting floor plan. Each wing was actually too narrow to provide proper corridor and room space. Moreover, the cramped corridors made the task of turning and manipulating guerneys or stretchers very difficult. The plan also limited any flexibility for future growth.

Following the years of legal disputes, the second hospital building was completed. On July 2, 1912, at seven-thirty in the morning, Archbishop Riordan celebrated a Pontifical Mass in the chapel of Mary's Help Hospital. The assistants were Fathers John J. Cantwell, Secretary to the Archbishop and future Archbishop of Los Angeles; P. J. Cummins, Chancellor of the Archdiocese; P. E. Mulligan, Secretary of the hospital Board; D. O. Crowley, President of the San Francisco Youth Directory; C. E. Kennedy, Assistant Pastor of St. Paul's Church; and T. J. Depta, C.M., Assistant Pastor of St. Vincent's Church, Los Angeles.

Patients were also admitted on that day. The first admission was Dr. A. P. O'Brien, President of the newly organized Medical Staff, who was hospitalized with a fractured leg. The second patient was a child from the Roman Catholic Orphanage. The hospital's first baby was also delivered on the morning of July 2, 1912 by Dr. Alexander Stanislaus "Pop" Keenan, who served as a member of the Board of the Corporation for 28 years and who, until his retirement in 1948, was known as "Mr. Mary's Help." This title was appropriate for Dr. Keenan, a prominent physician in San Francisco and tireless in his devotion to Mary's Help Hospital. He was one of the organizers of the Medical Staff and a friend of the student nurses.

Two Daughters of Charity had come to staff the hospital in 1910. During the construction they lived at O'Connor Hospital in San Jose and commuted to buy the equipment and furnishings for the new hospital. Ten Daughters of Charity were assigned to the hospital at the time of its opening. Sister Mary Angela O'Brien was the first Sister Servant and filled the role that is now called Administrator. Two Daughters of Charity had long years of uninterrupted service at Mary's Help Hospital from its opening in 1912 through its move in 1965. Sister Agatha Flynn, the first woman to be registered as a pharmacist in California, served in the Pharmacy and Clinic. Sister Ernestine Winiecke served in Maternity and was known throughout the hospital as the Sister who visited every patient in the hospital twice a day.

The Daughters of Charity at Mary's Help Hospital at the time of the 1912 dedication were:

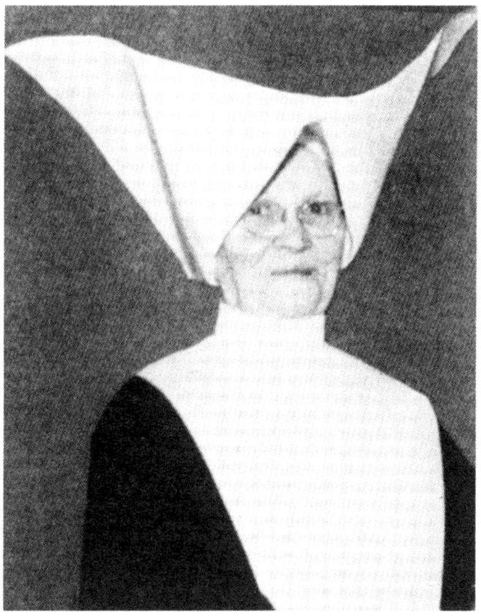

Sister Agatha Flynn.

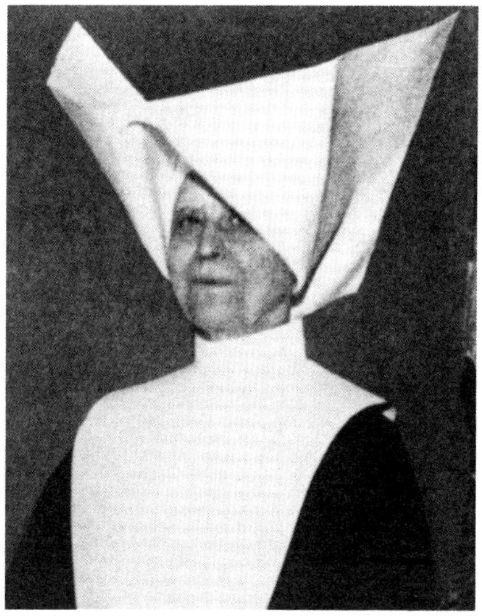

Sister Ernestine Winiecke.

Sister Mary Angela O'Brien
Sister Servant (Superior)*
Sister Elizabeth Bruen
Sister Irene Clark
Sister Ernestine Donnelly
Sister Juliana Donovan
Sister Agatha Flynn
Sister Emily Hannon
Sister Isadore Healy
Sister Martha Lawlor
Sister Ernestine Winiecke

In the same week of the dedication of Mary's Help Hospital, Archbishop Riordan also dedicated the rebuilt Roman Catholic Orphanage at 1700 Newhall Street in San Francisco. The original

*The title "Sister Servant" may be explained by the role reversal insisted upon by St. Vincent de Paul when he gave instructions to the Daughters of Charity in the care of the sick and the poor. The sick and the poor were to be the patrons; those offering the service were the servants, and as servers were to be enriched by the association. The Daughters of Charity refer to their Superior as Sister Servant.

building had been destroyed by fire in October of 1910. After the fire, the orphans were given shelter at the home of the Christian Brothers at Franklin and Ellis streets. When the new building was completed, 400 resident children were cared for there.

During this time the name of the orphanage was changed to Mount St. Joseph School. This third home of the Roman Catholic Orphan Asylum was vastly different from the first one at Market and Montgomery Streets. The first property had been deeded by Archbishop Joseph Sadoc Alemany in 1851. It was to this humble foundation of the system of Catholic Charities in California that the first Daughters of Charity came to San Francisco in 1852.

Following the establishment of the social agencies and schools, the Daughters of Charity in San Francisco began their third work—health care—when Mary's Help Hospital opened its doors in 1912.

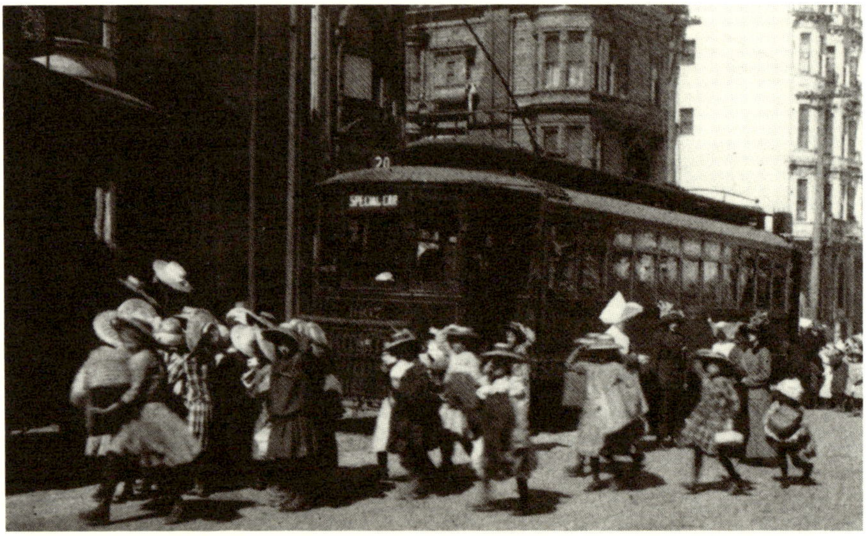

Moving the orphans to their new home at 1700 Newhall Street, San Francisco; July 1912.

Our Beginning as Mary's Help Hospital 1912–1920

THE MISSION OF MARY'S HELP HOSPITAL—to extend Christ's mission of healing in the spirit of St. Vincent de Paul —has been the driving force from our origin in 1912. The "small" hospital on the edge of the Mission District reached out to the people of San Francisco from its very beginning. Outstanding evidence of this dedication was seen in the quality of care provided, the School of Nursing and the Clinic services.

During the early years of Mary's Help Hospital "some Sisters, some doctors, some nurses" were all that were considered necessary to run a hospital efficiently. Along with a few lay workers, this was the hospital work force. Student nurses were responsible for many tasks and assignments that were not directly related to nursing care—for example, housekeeping and dietary duties. Despite the absence of a specialized clinical experience program and a curriculum that would be considered adequate by today's standards, Mary's Help School of Nursing prospered. Student nurses had the benefit and support of visionary Superintendents of Nurses, or Directors of Nursing as they were later called. It is a tribute to their work and foresight that our standards of excellence in nursing theory and practice were established and maintained.

The Articles of Incorporation of Mary's Help Hospital set forth some guidelines for the education of nurses:

> *Said Sisters of St. Vincent de Paul, under the direction and control of and as part of the work of Mary's Help Hospital, conduct and operate at and on said hospital premises a College of Nursing, commonly known and referred to as Mary's Help College of Nursing.*
>
> *The purpose for which said College of Nursing is operated and conducted is to carry on and maintain a training school for nurses*

for the purpose of training, teaching and educating nurses for the care and nursing of the sick and disabled, and for the purpose of teaching all sciences connected with the art of nursing, and to constitute chairs and to elect professors from the medical profession to teach such sciences and arts as are usually taught in schools and colleges for the training of nurses to care for the sick and disabled, to grant and at its will revoke and recall diplomas and medals, and to do all things necessary, desirable, or proper for such corporation to do in the promotion of its said objects.

Mary's Help was one of the first schools of nursing to be accredited by the California State Board of Nursing. The history of Mary's Help

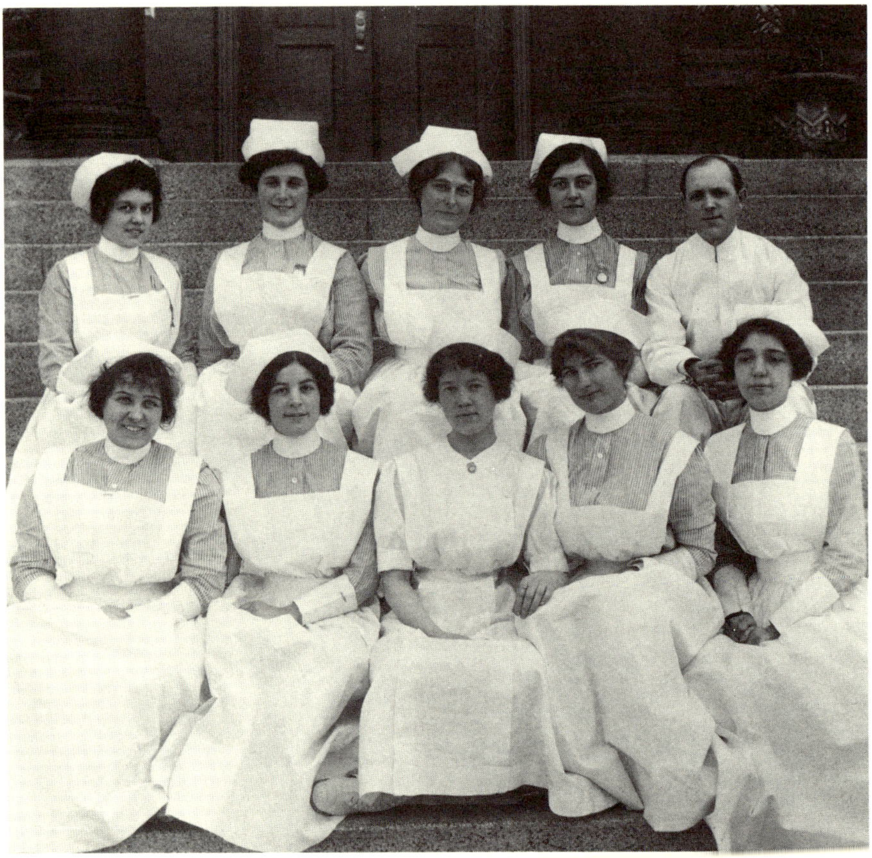

Members of the first graduating class, Mary's Help Hospital College of Nursing, 1914.

nurses is an extraordinary one. The graduates from 1914 to 1963, when the school was closed, were all part of a proud tradition. They form a group which has made significant contributions to all branches of nursing. It has become part of our heritage that one can recognize a Mary's Help Hospital nurse by her excellence of practice.

The first Superintendent of Nursing, Sister Martha Lawlor, was followed by Sister Dolores Carlos, who remained in that position until 1933. Their standards of appropriate practice and behavior for a Mary's Help nurse became the reference point for future generations of nurses. Sister Dolores is a legend in the memories of "her" nurses and the physicians who served in the early days of the hospital.

Members of the first graduating class of Mary's Help Hospital in 1914 were Elizabeth Ahern, Charles Allen, Edna Anderson, Alice Bretland, Ethel Gibney, Mary Gleese, Kathleen Kelleher, Felicia Taix, Anne Tiernan, and Dora Wernecke.

On September 7, 1912, a contract between the Corporation of Mary's Help Hospital and the Daughters of Charity was signed in agreement that the Daughters of Charity would manage, conduct, and maintain the hospital for a period of 50 years. Archbishop Patrick Riordan and Reverend Patrick Mulligan signed for the Corporation; Sister Eugenia Fealy, Visitatrix, and Sister Dolores Carlos signed for the Daughters of Charity. This document was prepared and filed by a San Francisco attorney named John J. O'Toole. It is worth noting here that his wife, Mrs. Christine O'Toole, was one of the first Presidents of the Mary's Help Hospital Guild as well as the sister of Sister Mary Barbara Regan of the Daughters of Charity.

On July 19, 1913, the feast of St. Vincent de Paul, the Outpatient Clinic opened. This free clinic was the first of its kind in the state. The event was noted in the *San Francisco Examiner*:

FUNDS NEEDED TO PAY FOR MEDICINES

The first Catholic free clinic in the State of California has just opened at Mary's Help Hospital in this city. Already, although but a few days in existence, it is proving popular and of greatest assistance to the public. The establishment of this free clinic has been contemplated for some time, but it was necessary to first place the hospital on such a financial footing that it could bear the extra expense incurred; and now Mary's Help offers the first free clinic opened by any Catholic hospital in the State. . . .

Mary's Help Free Clinic Auxiliary became the first Ladies Auxiliary and Guild of the hospital. Mrs. M. A. Tobin was President; Mrs. A. Loughborough, First Vice-president; and Mrs. A. P. O'Brien, Second Vice-president. Sister Angela was the Treasurer. In the Autumn and Winter of 1913, the Auxiliary sponsored a series of card parties at the St. Francis Hotel in San Francisco. This group was very successful in raising money to ease the financial burdens facing the Clinic. During the first year of operation 9,000 patients were treated in the Clinic.

This was the era of World War I, 1914 to 1918. Archbishop Hanna pledged to the United States Government the services of the Daughters of Charity and the other nursing sisterhoods in the area. The Sisters and staff of Mary's Help Hospital responded to the request of the government "that all should do their part." A number of physicians and eleven nurses served overseas with the American Expeditionary Forces. Four nurses were assigned to base hospitals in the United States.

In response to a request by Clara D. Noyes, Director of the Bureau of Nursing Service, the Daughters of Charity were authorized to organize and conduct classes in First Aid under the direction of the Pacific Division of the American Red Cross. These classes were offered for both nursing students and lay groups. Fifty members of the Ladies Sodality of Mission Dolores Church attended the first class taught at the hospital. Members of the family of Sister Anne Casey, known to generations of San Franciscans as Principal of St. Vincent's /Cathedral High School, were among the Sodalists enrolled in this first class.

At the request of the Committee for National Defense, the hospital was also selected to accommodate the United States Student Nurse Reserve candidates.

When the Sisters and members of the Ladies Guild learned that the soldiers who were waiting at Angel Island for transportation overseas

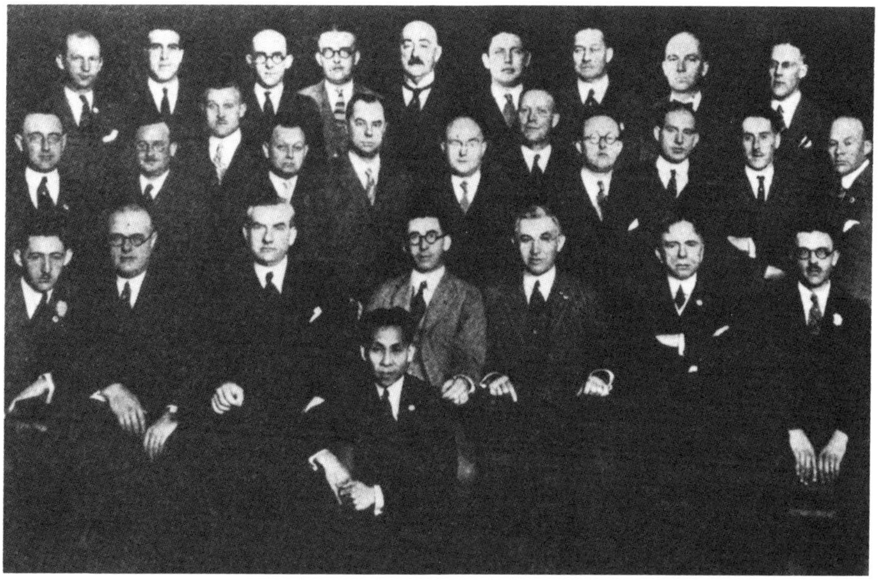

Medical and Surgical Staff, Mary's Help Hospital, San Francisco, 1920s.

had no Mass or chapel, they set up and equipped a chapel at the Angel Island Recruiting Station. Thereafter, Father John Rogers of St. Patrick's Church in San Francisco offered Mass each Sunday for the soldiers.

The nationwide influenza epidemic struck in the Fall of 1918; San Francisco was not spared. The number of new cases reached 700 per day and by October 1918, there were 6,691 cases. From September through December 1918, there were 445,000 deaths in the United States. The medical and nursing staffs of Mary's Help Hospital responded to the epidemic. In addition, Archbishop Hanna sent Christian Brothers and Holy Name Sisters to Mary's Help Hospital to help nurse the influenza victims. The hospital was licensed for 165 beds, but this number was increased to accommodate more patients. Every portion of available space was used for the influenza victims. It was said that even the space adjacent to the engine room was utilized for patients. The total number of influenza patients treated in-house was 774, while an additional 100 patients were nursed by Mary's Help Hospital staff in their homes.

Home care has always been an integral part of our services. Illustrating this is the following night letter sent to Sister Fidelis, Sister Servant of Mary's Help Hospital, from Sister Eugenia Fealy, Visitatrix, asking that Daughters of Charity from Mary's Help Hospital be sent to assist with the care of influenza patients in Menlo Park.

> NIGHT LETTER TO
>
> Sister Fidelis
Mary's Help Hospital
145 Guerrero St.
San Francisco, California
>
> If conditions have not improved at Menlo Park can you not send two sisters and then borrow from other houses to help you out. Sister Bruen says auto will be sent for sisters every morning and bring them back in evening. Have sisters wear masks, use spray and gargle.
>
> Marillac Seminary — *Sister Eugenia*
October 20, 1918 — 7:15 p.m.

St. Patrick's School became the home of the children whose mothers were influenza patients at Mary's Help Hospital. The Daughters of Charity cleared out the desks, set up beds, and supplied food and child care.

Hospital services grew rapidly during this period. As the services became more clearly defined and segregated, a Sister was assigned as supervisor of each area. Obstetrics, for example, became a separate service in 1917. The growth of this period was due in large part to the men who made up the original Medical Staff—to name a few, Doctors A. P. O'Brien, Alexander Keenan, A. A. O'Neill, T. D. Maher, Roderick O'Connor, A. T. Leonard, Vincent Derham, Charles Mohun, George Brady and I. W. Thorne, who was the nephew of Dr. W. S. Thorne, member of the original Board of Directors in 1893. Assisting the physicians was Hilario Marquez, Ph.D., who established and became Director of the Hospital Laboratory. These men were among the most illustrious physicians practicing in San Francisco. They created a standard of medical care that was outstanding both in relation to professional practice and to caring for the poor.

3

Our Time of Growth in San Francisco 1920–1930

SAN FRANCISCO experienced rapid growth and expansion during the twenties. With the completion of the Panama Canal, ships and commerce arriving from Europe and Asia made the San Francisco Harbor one of the busiest ports in the United States. The downtown business district expanded and created a critical need for housing. Builders transformed the sand dunes in the western portion of San Francisco into the residential districts of the Richmond and the Sunset. Early builders of the Sunset District and, later, Parkside and Twin Peaks were Carl and Fred Gellert, who along with their families have become major donors to the hospital. They established the Carl Gellert Foundation and the Fred Gellert Foundation as the means of continuing their gifts and philanthropy.

Mary's Help Hospital continued to work toward fulfilling its mission of providing health care services. Hospital admissions climbed steadily. Clinic services expanded. We began our work with the Catholic Hospital Association to upgrade standards for Catholic hospitals and Catholic nursing schools.

In the 1920s there were three Catholic hospitals in San Francisco: St. Mary's, sponsored by the Sisters of Mercy; St. Joseph's, sponsored by the Franciscan Sisters of the Sacred Heart; and Mary's Help—the only archdiocesan hospital—managed by the Daughters of Charity. Archbishop Riordan was succeeded in 1915 by Archbishop Edward Hanna, the third Archbishop of San Francisco. Archbishop Hanna was a friend of Mary's Help and made many visits to the hospital and, in particular, to the Clinic. San Franciscans remember him as a "great walker"; he was often seen walking down Clinton Park and entering the Clinic by the side door.

By this time the Clinic had expanded to offer a full range of services, including a Dental Clinic organized and staffed for many years by Dr.

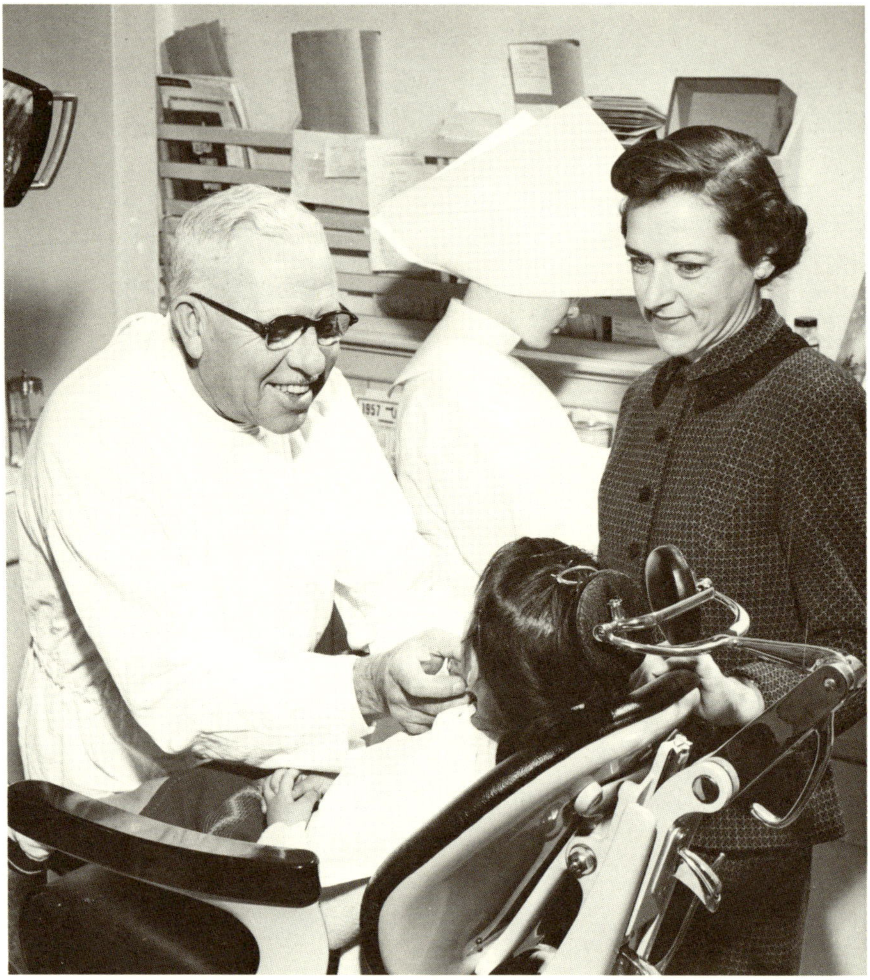

Dr. Paul Gilbert (1957), who organized the dental clinic in 1923.

Paul Gilbert. In 1923, there were 18,136 Clinic visits and an additional 361 home visits. There were also 4,627 inpatient admissions to the hospital that same year.

The hospital's Maternity Service grew very rapidly during this period. Sister Fidelis Ryan, the second Sister Servant and Administrator, saw the need to provide a facility for unwed mothers. To this end, in 1921 Archbishop Hanna made possible the first St. Elizabeth's

Hospital, located in what had been an old-fashioned mansion on Van Ness Avenue and Filbert Street. Dr. John McQuade of the Mary's Help Hospital Medical Staff directed the provision of medical care at St. Elizabeth's Hospital. The need for this service continued, and in 1928 the Bartholomew P. Oliver family, long-time patrons of the work of the Daughters of Charity, built and helped endow the new St. Elizabeth's Hospital at 100 Masonic Avenue. In 1977, St. Elizabeth's was consolidated with Mount St. Joseph's, which provides group homes for teenage girls. The Daughters of Charity have served for 64 years at St. Elizabeth's and 133 years at Mount St. Joseph's. Another name to be remembered for long service to St. Elizabeth's is Dr. Andrew M. Ryan, a Mary's Help obstetrician. He directed the medical care at St. Elizabeth's for many years.

During this period, nursing followed the example of medicine in critically examing the educational standards of hospital schools of nursing. The Flexner Report, published in 1910, prompted organized medicine to inaugurate a system of academic standards that greatly reduced the number of medical schools and improved the quality of medical education. A few years later, the Rockefeller Foundation financed a comparable study of nursing education. The study was directed by Dr. C. A. Winslow of Yale University and Josephine Goldmark, for whom the study was named. The Goldmark Report, "Nursing, and Nursing Education in the United States," published in 1923, was critical of the standards of many hospital-sponsored schools of nursing. Unlike the Flexner Report, which had a major impact on medical education, the Goldmark Report did not establish national uniform standards of nursing education. However, the records at Mary's Help reveal that great attention was paid to the recommendations and findings of this report. The Goldmark Report was used at Mary's Help as strong support for maintaining high standards of nursing education.

In 1921, Sister Zoe Schiezwold replaced Sister Fidelis as Sister Servant and Administrator. In 1927, Sister Zoe was replaced by Sister Regina Maloney. During Sister Regina's administration the Depression made tremendous demands upon the Daughters, the hospital,

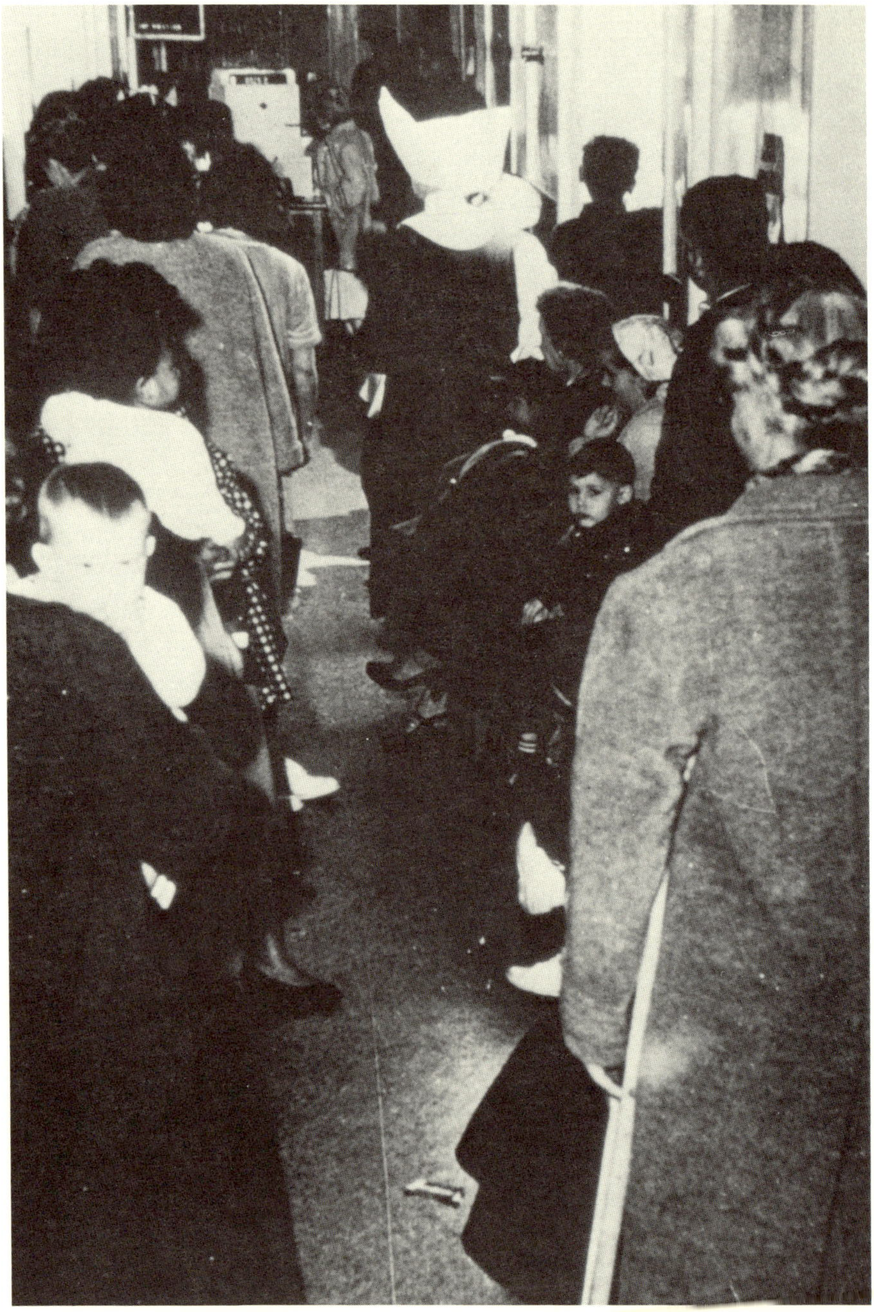

Patients waiting to be seen in the free clinic, Mary's Help Hospital, San Francisco.

and, in particular, the Clinic. The ratio of free-care and part-pay patients to those who were able to pay for care was more than two to one. In addition to providing inpatient and clinic services to the needy, the hospital fed the hungry who came to Mary's Help every day. In 1929, there were 8,836 Clinic patients. Records show that 36,585 meals and 5,900 free prescriptions were given to the poor. The Sisters and nurses made 2,333 home visits to supply food, clothing, and medicine.

Seeing the Sisters and nurses care for the poor is one of my earliest memories of Mary's Help Hospital. I remember walking down Guerrero Street on my way to school and seeing Brosnan Street, a small street to the left of the hospital, filled with men standing shoulder to shoulder. They were there every morning at 8:00 a.m.—waiting. At noon when I came home for lunch, there was always a Sister and some nurses serving food and hot soup. This went on day after day. Actually, years later when I was a student nurse at the hospital and realized how poor the hospital was, I wondered how the Sisters had fed so many people for so long. The poor were always cared for at Mary's Help.

Ninety-eight student nurses graduated from the Mary's Help School of Nursing from 1920 to 1930. Three became members of religious orders. Genevieve McArdle was one of the three; she became Sister Genevieve McArdle of the Daughters of Charity and returned to serve at Mary's Help Hospital many years later.

Nurses were a very important part of the hospital's work force during this period. The nursing program was a twenty-eight week basic course followed by eight months of advanced courses. The additional eight months proved to be a wise requirement because the State of California later passed a law requiring that nursing education programs be three years in length. Mary's Help nurses also had an academic advantage when they applied for college entrance to further their nursing education. The theoretical and practical curricula are listed on the next page.

MARY'S HELP HOSPITAL NURSING PROGRAM

Arrangement of Course of Theory

Preparatory Period (16 Weeks)

Anatomy and Physiology	32 hours
Bacteriology	8 hours
Personal Hygiene	8 hours
Applied Chemistry	16 hours
Nutrition and Cooking (2-hour periods)	32 hours
Nursing Procedures (including bandaging)	64 hours
Drugs and Solutions	16 hours
Ethics of Nursing	8 hours

First Junior Session (16 Weeks)

Anatomy and Physiology	16 hours
Medical Nursing (including diseases of the skin)	16 hours
Materia Medica	16 hours
Diet in Disease	8 hours
Surgical Nursing	8 hours

Second Junior Session (16 Weeks)

Surgical Nursing (including Orthopedics and Gynecology)	12 hours
Operating Room Technique	10 hours
Clinical Pathology, Urinalysis and Laboratory Technique	15 hours
Communicable Diseases (including Tuberculosis and Venereal Diseases)	12 hours
Eye, Ear, Nose and Throat	8 hours

First Senior Session (16 Weeks)

Obstetrical Nursing	16 hours
Pediatrics (including Infant Feeding)	16 hours
Mental and Nervous Diseases	8 hours

Second Senior Session (16 Weeks)

Hygiene and Public Sanitation	8 hours
History and Development of Nursing	8 hours
Private Duty Nursing	4 hours

Introduction to Branches of Nursing

Public Health Nursing	2 hours
Administrative Work	2 hours
Instructor's Work	2 hours

Practical Work

General Medical Nursing	6 months
Surgical Nursing	6 months
Obstetrical Nursing	3 months
Care of Sick Children	3 months
Infant Care	3 months
Diet Kitchen	2 months
Operating Room	3 months

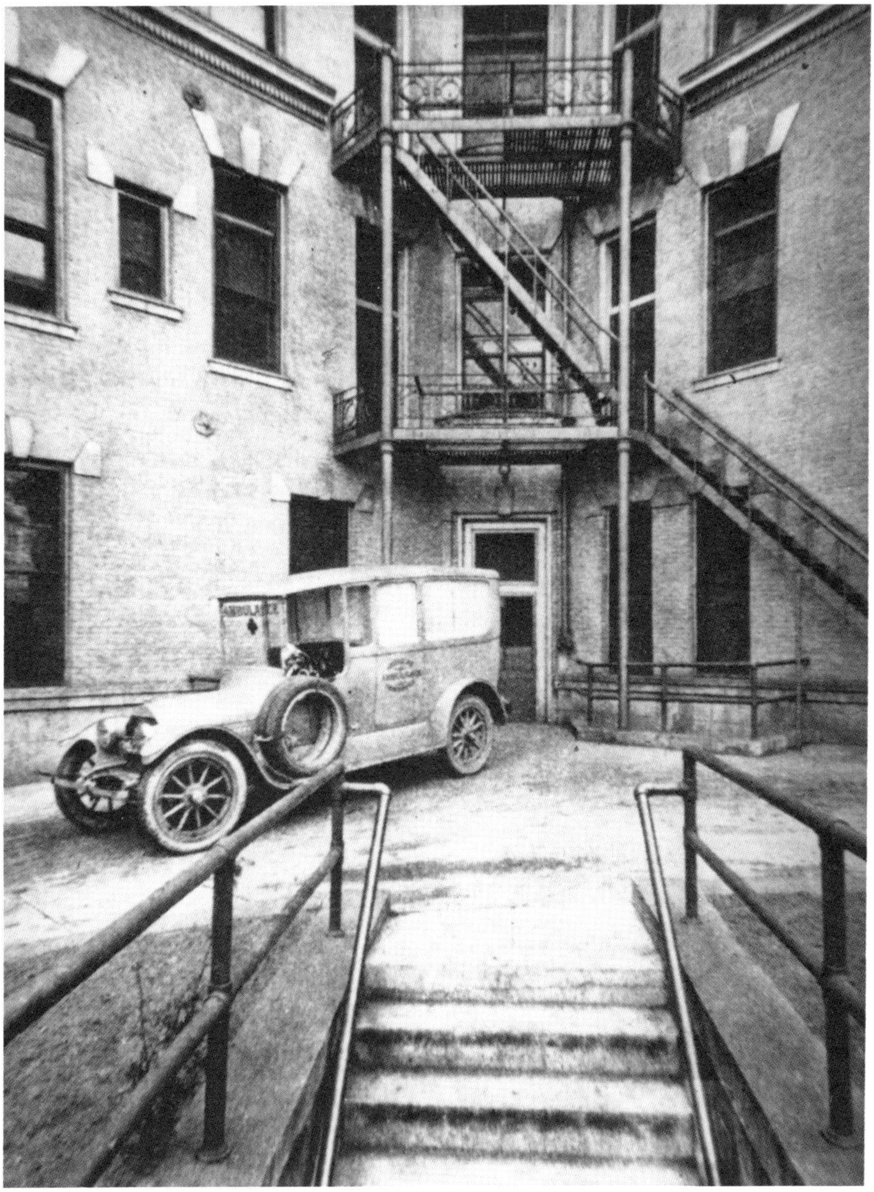

Ambulance waiting at the Emergency entrance, Mary's Help Hospital, 1925.

In this period, several employees joined us for what became long terms of service. Raymonda Dawson established the Social Services Department in the Clinic. Grace Bruneman O'Hanlon joined the Business Department, where she remained for forty years. It was Grace who negotiated so successfully with the Community Chest (now the United Way) for funds for the Clinic and hospital. The annual allotment from the Community Chest was always eagerly awaited by the hospital staff, because it was critical in maintaining the Clinic, and part-pay and free hospitalization. Grace retired in December 1967. Her career was noteworthy for her loyal support of the Sisters and the hospital.

The practice of admitting patients on a long-term basis was not unusual at that time. Mrs. Nellie McKenna was an arthritic with deformities that made her unable to care for herself. She was a patient for thirty-three years. Although she was physically limited, mentally and emotionally she was a giant and a friend to all at Mary's Help Hospital. Miss Mary Lee, a veteran employee of the diet kitchen, retired to a room on the second surgical floor and used it as her home. Sixteen years later when she became ill, she was cared for until her death there.

The years 1920 to 1930 were times of expansion and growth both for San Francisco and the hospital. However, at the end of the decade, the deepening Depression created new problems.

4

The Depression Years 1930–1940

THE THIRTIES INCREASED THE DEMANDS on Mary's Help Hospital for clinic services, and free and part-pay hospitalization. Sister Agatha was in charge of the Clinic and Pharmacy during this period. Through practice and example she inspired the entire staff of the hospital to follow her in her truly Vincentian administration of charity.

The *San Francisco Examiner* on September 12, 1931 described some of the hospital's charity work:

> *This "Monument of Faith" in the Archdiocese of San Francisco, not only caters to the needs of the sick, but cares for the poor and unemployed. A feature of the hospital is its bread line and free clinic. The Sisters serve an average of over 10,000 free meals each month, and take care of thousands of sick each year, who are unable to pay for medicine or medical attention.*

The physicians were very devoted to Sister Agatha and to the Clinic. Outpatient services, provided by members of the Medical Staff in all specialties, continued to expand. Hospital patients who were unable to pay were cared for as well. While all the names of the physicians are not recorded here, some of the doctors I can recall from this period were Hans von Geldern and Andrew Ryan in Obstetrics and Gynecology; Isaac Walton Thorne, Alexander Stanislaus "Pop" Keenan and Everett Carlson in Surgery; Alfred C. Reed and Francis Rochex in Internal Medicine; Dudley Smith in Proctology; Merrill Mensor and Leon Parker in Orthopedics; Victor McPhee and Ben Hagan in Pediatrics; Zera Bolin in Pathology; Fredrick Rodenbaugh in Radiology; William Joseph Crawford in Ophthalmology; and Henry Gardner, Arthur Vollert and John Henry Golden in General Medicine.

There are many people who gave generously of their time and talents to help the sick at Mary's Help. In 1934, there were 9,801 Clinic patients, 16,101 Clinic visits, and 725 home visits. The people of San

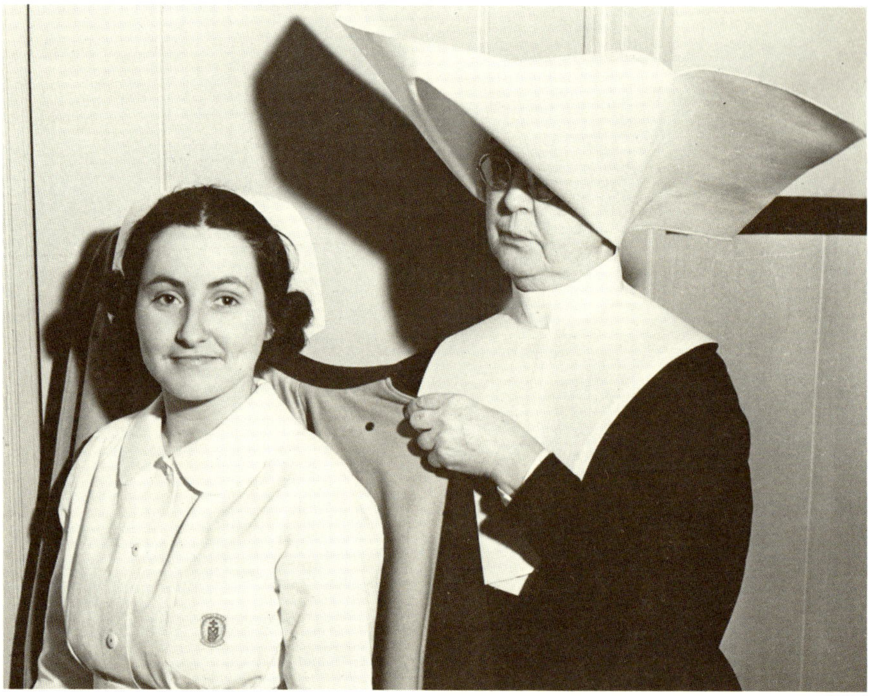

Sister Stephanie Wall, Superintendent of Nurses, at a capping ceremony with one of her student nurses, late 1930s.

Francisco remembered the charity dispensed at the hands of the Daughters of Charity at 145 Guerrero Street in later years when the fund drives for the hospital were held.

In 1933, Sister Regina was replaced by Sister Fidelis Ryan, who returned for her second term as Sister Servant and Administrator. Sister Fidelis served until her death in 1939.

Also in 1933, Sister Dolores, the Superintendent of Nurses, was replaced by Sister Stephanie Wall. Sister Dolores had established an enviable reputation as an excellent nursing educator. The dedication of her Mary's Help nurses to professional nursing was well recognized in San Francisco and throughout California. Sister Stephanie was also a nursing leader. Sister was the person in charge of nursing when I was a student nurse; as it was she who directed me into nursing education, I believe I am permitted a few reminiscences.

Sister Stephanie was born in Lynchburg, Virginia, and from her point of view the Civil War was an unfinished chapter. As her students, we became loyal supporters of the Confederacy because on Robert E. Lee's birthday there was a general late leave. This was no small favor since our days were filled with long hours of duty and classes. Late leaves to 11:15 p.m. were issued one per month and were very easily forfeited or rescinded.

Sister Stephanie felt her student nurses should be educated in fields other than nursing. We enrolled in economics classes at Dominican College in San Rafael and in parliamentary law classes at Lone Mountain in San Francisco. Sister also noticed that many of the fifteen student nurses in her first class did not stand erect and had poor posture. She then contracted with the Presidio, and an officer came at 6:30 a.m. on weekdays for drill practice. We later recognized Sister Stephanie's visionary leadership—however reluctant we were at times to accept her mandates!

We were introduced to a variety of topics in addition to an excellent nursing program. Sister Stephanie, who had been a pharmacist in the Spanish-American War, had an interest which never waned in *materia medica*, as pharmacology was then called. We were well-prepared in this subject, and indeed, obtaining those precious late leaves was contingent upon passing the weekly Friday night examinations. Sister Stephanie was a true leader—one who inspired and encouraged us to grow and strive beyond normal limits as nurses and also as Christian women. Her influence will not be forgotten.

At the same time, Francis Curry, brother of Sister Carmel Curry of the Daughters of Charity, was a friend to the nurses. He was a medical student working on the switchboard at night, and was always helpful to the students who returned a bit late. After graduation from medical school, Dr. Curry directed the San Francisco Public Health Department. In retirement now, he directs St. Anthony's Medical Clinic, a free service for the poor.

On June 10, 1934, in honor of the canonization of St. Louise de Marillac, co-foundress of the Daughters of Charity, there was a

Solemn Pontifical Mass offered by Monsignor Charles A. Ramm at St. Mary's Cathedral on Van Ness Avenue. Archbishop Edward J. Hanna was also present. The homilist was Father Martin J. Malley, C.M. The choir was composed of student nurses under the direction of Father Edgar Boyle, the Archdiocesan Director of Music. In the evening there was Benediction. Archbishop Hanna was the celebrant and Father Thomas C. Powers, the homilist.

In 1936, the hospital welcomed its first resident chaplain, Father Mark Lappen, from Denver. Prior to this time, the patients were visited by the priests from the nearby Mission Dolores Church. Daily Mass at 5:30 a.m. was offered by Father Pius, O.F.M., who walked to Mary's Help each morning from St. Boniface Church on Golden Gate Avenue.

The hospital was busy in this decade. The Medical Staff was

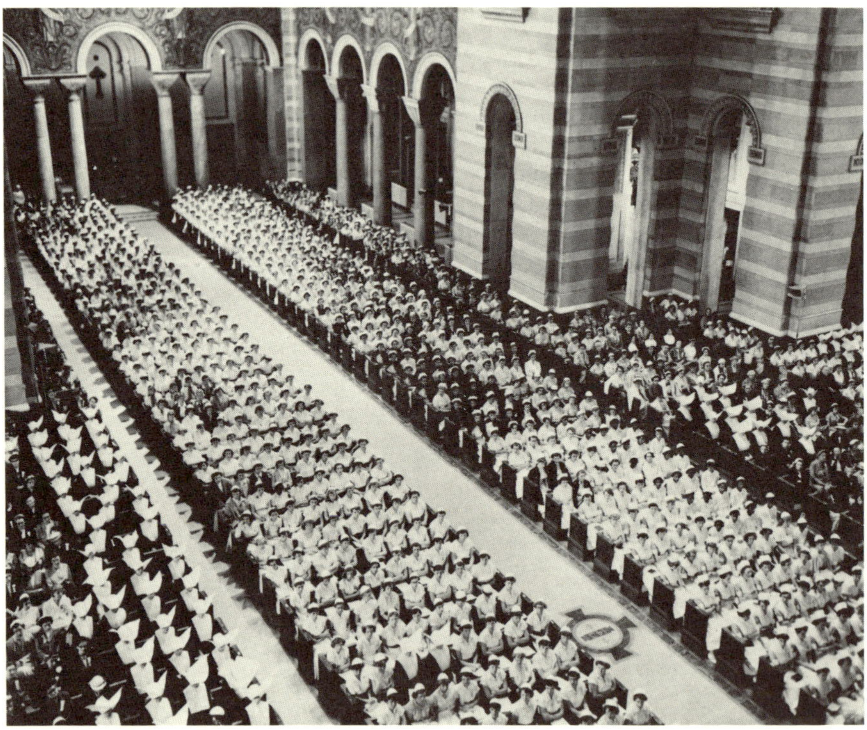

Solemn Pontifical Mass for the canonization of St. Louise de Marillac, St. Mary's Cathedral, San Francisco, June 10, 1934.

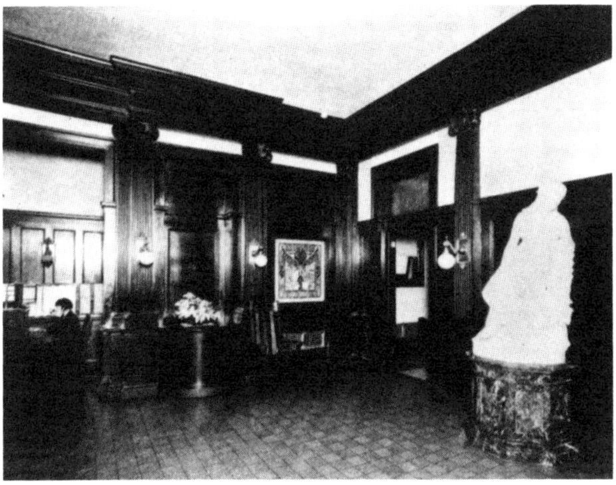

The Promised Land statue in the front lobby of old Mary's Help Hospital, San Francisco.

growing, and 163 nurses, including three Daughters of Charity, graduated from the School of Nursing. They included Sister Lucia Sheehy in 1932, Sister Martina Foley in 1933, and Sister Mary Jane Breidenbach in 1934.

In 1939, Sister Fidelis, who is remembered for her unfailing kindness and gentle manner, died suddenly of a stroke. Sister Basil Thyken came from St. Thomas Hospital in Nashville to be Sister Servant and Administrator of Mary's Help Hospital.

In the late thirties, a large marble statue called *The Promised Land* (the figure was reputed to be Miriam, sister of Moses) was removed from the lobby and placed in the courtyard. Sister Basil made this major decision when she decided to begin remodeling the hospital lobby. Representatives of the Medical Staff, led by Dr. Keenan, were present to insure that the moving process would be carried out correctly and that the courtyard was suitable for this very important part of Mary's Help Hospital. Relocation was actually a difficult task. The statue was large and heavy, and transporting it down the front steps to Brosnan Street and into the courtyard was not easy. As a representative of the nursing students assigned to be present, it was my thought that these workmen may well have decided to give up the moving business for another line of work after this assignment. I am sure they never experienced so many instructions and directions as to how they should do their work as they received on that day!

At the close of this decade, the hospital's "Emergency Service" was established when construction of the Bay and Golden Gate Bridges was in progress. Staff physicians including Doctors Merrill Mensor, Leon Parker and LaRue Moore had contracts with insurance companies to care for injured bridge workers. Many patients were brought to the treatment room, as it was then called. It was located on the second floor of the hospital near the men's ward and staffed by personnel from Central Supply, which was on the third floor. The notification system was a simple one—nurses in Central Supply, on the third floor, were verbally summoned by the second floor nurses when a patient arrived. This system was replaced in April, 1940 when a telephone was installed in the treatment room. After initial treatment many of the patients with orthopedic injuries were hospitalized with us for long periods of time. My first position after graduation was as treatment room nurse for the bridge workers.

5

The War Years and Changes 1940–1950

DURING THE FORTIES we focused our energies on a major concern—remodeling of the hospital. However, the events of December 7, 1941—bringing the United States into World War II—obscured the importance of any other priorities.

In the early part of 1940, before the war began, Sister Basil began her renovations. The lobby, admitting office, and main corridor were completely renovated. A beautiful red, tan, and green terrazzo floor was constructed. The old switchboard at the front door was replaced by a new executone system. Offices were remodeled, and two guest rooms were added. A new fire alarm system was installed. It was the first alarm system connected to both the central system and the San Francisco Fire Department. New fire extinguishers were also placed throughout the hospital. The extinguisher in the visitors' waiting room was put to immediate and successful use to extinguish a fire in the palm tree in the maternity courtyard.

The history of Mary's Help Hospital and of union negotiations goes back to our beginnings in San Francisco. However, the first real test of our relations with the unions took place in June, 1940. The members of the Hospital and Institutional Workers Union had announced that they would call a strike on June 19. But early that morning, representatives of the union told Sister Basil that neither the membership nor public opinion would support a strike against Mary's Help Hospital. The work of the hospital was a vital part of the day-to-day life of the community.

On September 9, 1941, the hospital received national publicity. The first person to jump from the recently completed Golden Gate Bridge and to survive became a patient at Mary's Help Hospital. Dr. Merrill C. Mensor, Chief of the Division of Orthopedics, was the surgeon who treated the woman's fractured back and reconstructed her arm and hand. She was a patient for eight months and had a complete recovery.

When she was first admitted, the hospital had to employ extra help to handle the phone calls, mail and gifts arriving for her.

The remodeling of the hospital continued. The doctors' lounge and the nurses' quarters on the fourth and fifth floors were redone. As always, the Guild was helpful in the renovation projects. On December 4, 1941, the Guild organized a very successful Charity Race Day at Tanforan Race Track for the benefit of Mary's Help Hospital and the British War Relief.

Three days later the United States was at war. On December 8, 1941, a representative from the Twelfth Naval District asked how many beds could be made available for wounded Navy patients. That same day the Medical Staff met to organize their services to care for possible air-raid victims. The police came at 7:10 p.m. and ordered a black-out of the entire hospital. Drapes and shutters were erected. The service of the hospital continued without interruption.

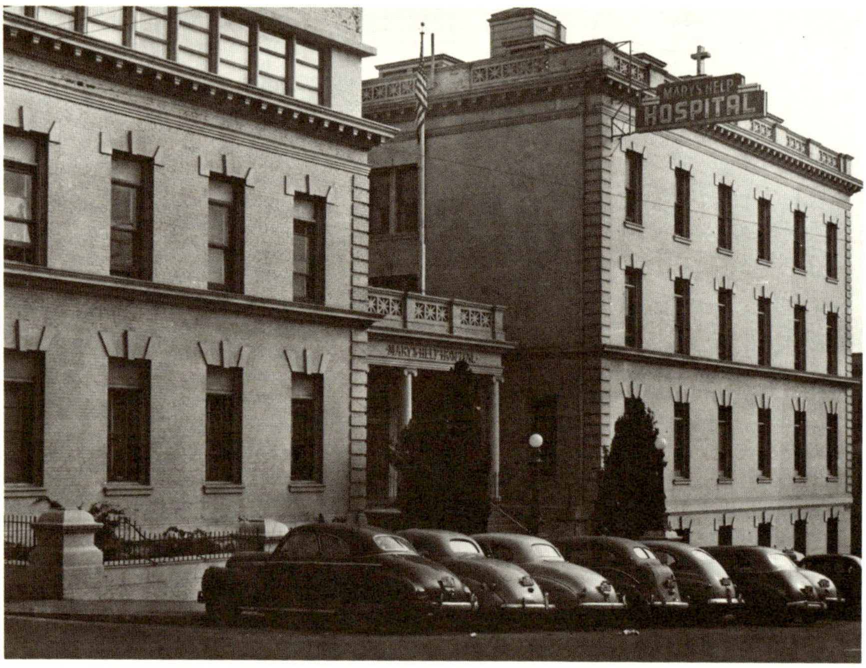

Mary's Help Hospital after the addition of the new maternity wing on the roof of the old Annex building.

The war brought many changes and shortages. Physicians, nurses and other personnel left for the service. As the number of patients increased, the shortage of space available for patient care became a major concern. These changes, along with the nightly black-outs and air-raid sirens, made life at 145 Guerrero Street very different.

Early in the war, officers of the Twelfth Naval District approached Sister Basil with the request to use Mary's Help as an auxiliary hospital for the wives of servicemen for obstetrical care. We had a busy Maternity Service, but this addition made it a burgeoning one. The Navy supplied their own medical officers and physicians, who were on duty around the clock. By 1944 the number of Navy births became so great that a new maternity wing was built on the roof of the old annex building. New delivery rooms and nurseries were constructed. The old delivery room and nursery were converted to much-needed patient rooms.

Our wartime service to the Navy was recognized at a civic ceremony on July 27, 1948. Captain James J. O'Connor, U.S.N., presented a certificate of appreciation to Sister Alphonsa, Hospital Administrator, for the Daughters of Charity:

> *For their sincere personal service and patient unselfish interest far exceeding the normal care of patients. The Sisters frequently visited the sick and assisted materially as well as spiritually in the recovery of all patients.*

A Meritorious Certificate of Achievement was presented to the hospital:

> *For outstanding service to the Navy Medical Department during the war years far exceeding the normal care of patients.*

Our chaplain, Father Thomas Scahill, accepted the certificate and responded for Archbishop Mitty and the Daughters of Charity:

> *On behalf of His Excellency, our Most Reverend Archbishop, and on behalf of the Daughters of Charity of St. Vincent de Paul, the members of the Board of Directors, and the entire hospital staff, it is my happy privilege to extend a deep expression of gratitude to the United States Navy on this lovely occasion of the presentation of these citations of merit to our dearly beloved Sisters and Mary's Help Hospital.*

We are deeply conscious of the singular honor which our grateful government has seen fit to confer upon us.

During war, great sacrifices must needs be demanded from every group, from every citizen in the nation. The Sisters, ever mindful of this, were only too eager to give of the very best they could offer by way of service on the homefront.

Anyone conversant with the story of the Daughters of Charity will remember their contributions to mankind in peace and in war. While the modern profession of nursing originates through the efforts of Florence Nightingale, it is well to remember that she received her inspiration and training from the Daughters of Charity in Paris. Need anyone mention the glory of the Medical Corps in the late war. It is axiomatic that they rendered service both valuable and intelligent. It remains for me to express to Captain O'Connor of the U.S. Navy our gratitude to him for presiding on this occasion. We ask him to channel our thanks and abiding devotion to the proper authorities with an assurance of our loyalty to the country of our love.

Doctor Everett Carlson, a member of the Board of Directors of the Corporation, accepted the certificate for the hospital:

On behalf of the Board of Directors and the medical staff of Mary's Help Hospital, the purpose of this meeting is to honor the Sisters of this hospital for their contribution to the war effort.

It was through their endeavors that the facilities were created for the use of which the Navy is now bestowing upon them and this hospital this evidence of their appreciation.

The medical staff is very much gratified that the Daughters of Charity should receive this recognition.

In behalf of Archbishop Mitty's office, under whose direction these activities are conducted, I have been asked to accept the award to the hospital and to express thanks to Captain O'Connor, Admiral Swanson and the Navy Department for their fine gesture.

It is regrettable that some of the Sisters who did so much are not here today to receive the thanks they so richly deserve. Sister Basil, our Superior at that time, was tireless in her efforts to improve and enlarge the hospital. Sister Claire Toups, who then had charge of the maternity wing, carried an extraordinary burden. Her constant devotion to duty contributed so much to the proper care of the families of the Navy personnel. They deserve much credit.

I wish to take this opportunity to thank all the Sisters, the nursing staff, the operating room staff and anesthetists, and the technical staff for the fine work they did that brought this recognition to this hospital.

The Navy doctors who were assigned here were skillful doctors and fine gentlemen. We enjoyed their stay with us.

This hospital can well be proud of its contribution of medical personnel to both the Navy and the Army. I wish to pay my respects to you of the staff who went so willingly, served so ably, and achieved such a glorious victory. I'm afraid we are too prone to forget the sacrifices you made.

Since the Army is so well represented by Colonel John McGuinness, President of our Medical Staff, I think it would be fitting to hear from Captain Merrill Mensor of the Navy, who I believe is our ranking Naval representative.

Again, on behalf of the hospital and his Excellency Archbishop John J. Mitty, I wish to thank you, Captain O'Connor, for this award.

The wartime growth of the obstetrical service, the new obstetrical facilities, and the leadership of Dr. Chester Cooley made our Maternity Service outstanding. Dr. Cooley also developed an accredited residency program in Obstetrics and Gynecology. Dr. Hubert Schwarz was the first full-time resident. He later became Chairman of the Department of Obstetrics and Gynecology and President of the Medical Staff. Other members of this program who remain in active practice at the hospital are: Dr. Norman Wheeler, who served as Chairman of the Department of Obstetrics and Gynecology; Dr. Paul Fraser, former President of the Medical/Dental Staff; Dr. Frank Kmak, former President of the Medical/Dental Staff and present Chairman of the Department of Obstetrics and Gynecology; and Dr. Harold Torkelson, who, during his residency, wrote one of the early studies on the use of saddle-block anesthesia, which was pioneered at Mary's Help Hospital in 1949.

The Depression and the war created a national shortage of nurses and had a major impact upon the College of Nursing. In 1943, the U.S. Cadet Nurse Corps was established under the provision of the Nurse Training Act. It passed on June 15, 1943, to expand nursing education and prepare professional nurses.

The Nurse Training Act made many provisions for student nurses as indicated in this passage from the United States Public Health Service Bulletin Form 40:

> *Students who are members of the United States Cadet Nurse Corps, will have all tuition and fees paid by the United States Public Health Service as well as the uniforms and books provided. In addition, these students will receive stipends, for personal expenses of $15.00 a month for the first nine months, and $20.00 a month for the remainder of their clinical course.*
>
> *Membership in the Corps is purely voluntary on the part of the student. Upon admission to the Corps, any student and her parents should understand that the application for membership in the United States Cadet Nurse Corps constitutes a pledge to remain in nursing, in either civilian or military service, health permitting, throughout the war; requires the signature of the student's parents or legal guardian, if she has not reached the age of majority under state law.*
>
> *Federal aid will be continued, after the war, for completion of programs of students who have been enrolled in the Corps for at least ninety days prior to cessation of hostilities.*
>
> *Mothers and fathers of prospective students should be reassured that membership in the Corps does not mean that their daughters will be pressed into military service against their will.*

As a result the tempo of life in the College of Nursing quickened. Numbers of matriculating students were larger, and it was recommended that the hospital accept applicants more frequently and then combine them into one class at graduation. From 1944 to 1945, four groups were admitted in thirteen months.

Students and faculty members were issued uniforms of the Cadet Corps. They consisted of grey flannel suits, white blouses, grey flannel topcoats, grey raincoats, and grey felt berets. The uniforms were

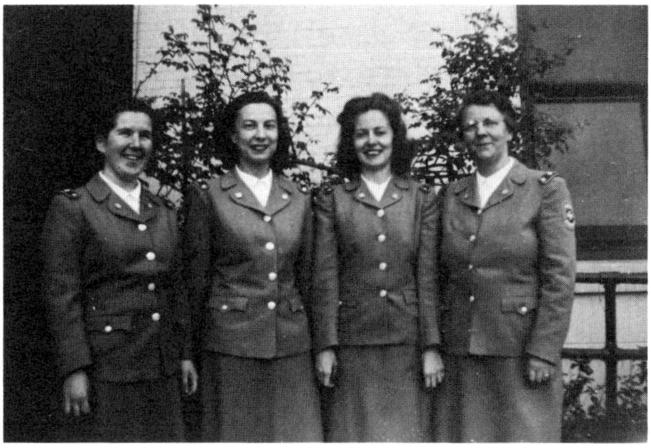

Mary's Help College of Nursing faculty members in the uniforms of the United States Cadet Nurse Corps.

trimmed with red epaulets. The sterling silver buttons and pins on the epaulets, designed by Tiffany's of New York, were inscribed with the caduceus, the Corps insignia.

The students and faculty of the College of Nursing—because of their participation in the United States Nurse Corps—were invited to attend sessions of the United Nations Conference, which opened in San Francisco on April 25, 1945.

The thirty-six-month program was condensed to thirty months. An additional six months were spent studying either at the School of Nursing or at Federal hospitals, the choice of which included Army, Navy, Marine, United States Public Health Service, Veteran's Administration, or Indian Service. The most popular choice among Mary's Help students was the Oak Knoll Naval Hospital in Oakland, where the faculty were also sent, as clinical instructors.

It was at the Oak Knoll Naval Hospital that I experienced both military regulations and the creative ingenuity of the servicemen. One day as we were preparing for the traditional white glove inspection of the ward by the ranking Admiral, we discovered that one of the two ward shower rooms was missing one of its two required curtains. This would be a serious problem in the inspection. However, we learned that the Navy would not issue a new shower curtain until we submitted the old one. It was not to be found. Finally, a very young sailor suggested that since the ward had two entrances with a shower room at each, we could hang two curtains in one shower, and then

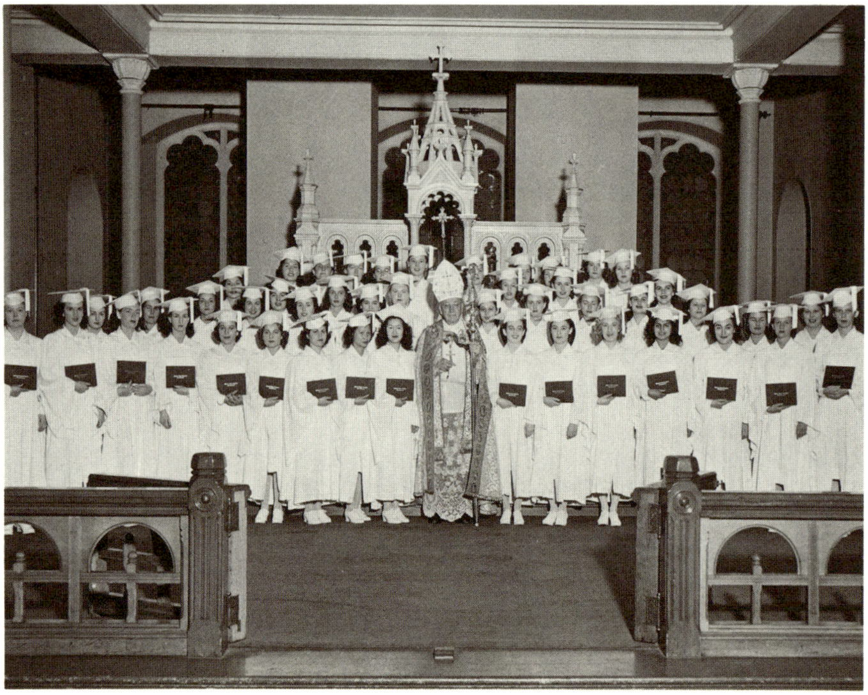

Archbishop John J. Mitty conferring diplomas on 45 new graduates of the class of 1947, the largest group to graduate from the College of Nursing.

while the inspection was going on he could remove one of them and put it in the second shower. The only problem was that no one knew which door the Admiral would enter. We decided to take the chance and hope for the best. It worked. The Admiral entered the right door and saw the shower room in perfect order with two curtains. By the time he reached the other shower, it also had two curtains!

The provisions of federal funds prompted more women to prepare as nurses. By 1945 the number of nursing students in the United States had rebounded from its Depression-era low of 67,533 to over 126,000 students.

During this period, Mary's Help offered six rotating internships for physicians. The service on each of these internships usually consisted of four months on General Medicine; four months on General Surgery

—including the surgical subspecialties; two months on Obstetrics and Gynecology; and two months on Pediatrics and Clinic. The Clinic included thirty-two medical/surgical outpatient services with fifty specialists participating in the Clinic program and in the interns' teaching program.

Residencies were offered in General Medicine, Surgery, Obstetrics and Gynecology. These were two-year programs and were approved by their respective specialty boards.

On February 28, 1946, the Articles of Incorporation of Mary's Help Hospital were amended, and the original fifty-year term of existence of the Corporation was made perpetual. Signing for the Corporation were Archbishop John J. Mitty, President; John A. Lally, Secretary; Alexander S. Keenan, M.D.; and John H. Golden, M.D.

In 1945, Sister Alphonsa Alcoin replaced Sister Basil as Sister Servant and Administrator. Sister Alphonsa continued the renovation program put in motion by Sister Basil. Two apartment buildings on Brosnan Street were purchased and modernized. The College of Nursing and student residences were all relocated there. The fourth and fifth floors of the hospital, former student residences, were modernized and became the medical wing of the hospital. In 1946, Congress passed the Hill-Burton Act, which provided funds for

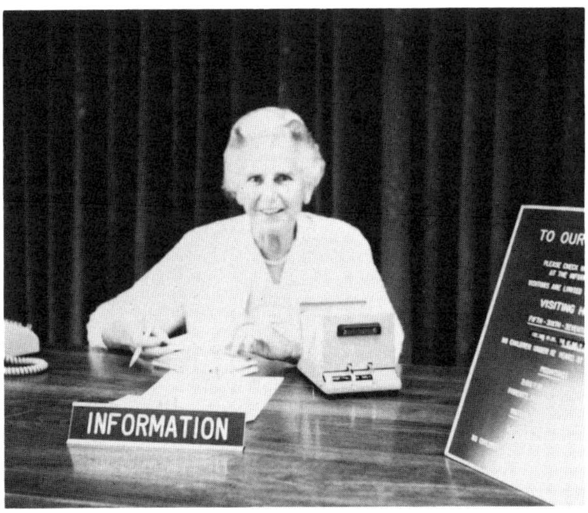

DR. PHILLIS BOURNE
First President of the reorganized Guild.

hospital construction. This legislation was very significant to us in the following two decades.

At the suggestion of Sister Alphonsa, the Guild was reorganized in 1950. The name was changed from the Saint Louise de Marillac Guild to the Mary's Help Hospital Guild. The first President of the new group was Doctor Phillis Bourne. The first project of the reorganized Guild was fund-raising for modernization of the operating room.

Two hundred and forty-one nurses graduated from 1940 to 1950. Ann McGuinn, a 1942 graduate, is now Sister Ann McGuinn of the Sisters of Saint Joseph of Orange and President of the Queen of the Valley Hospital in Napa, California.

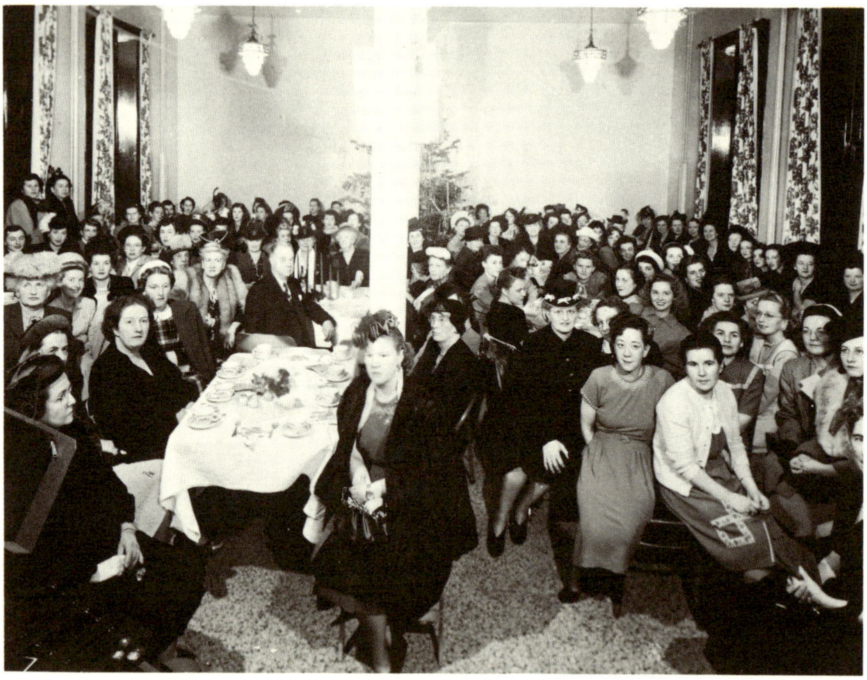

Mary's Help Hospital Nurses Alumnae Christmas Party, 1947;
Dr. Alexander S. Keenan, guest speaker.

6

The Years of Decision 1950–1960

THE DECADE FROM 1950 TO 1960 reflected the continued dynamism of life at Mary's Help. We experienced a full range of emotions, including sorrow, fear and joy. On the one hand, we lost several dear friends, and an earthquake damaged the hospital in 1957. On the other hand, we took pride in being recognized by the community for our service. Through all the happy and sad events that affected Mary's Help Hospital, it also became clear to us that the time for major change had come.

The decade had a very sad beginning for us. Sister Ambrose Fox, Sacristan and Supervisor of Surgery, was killed. She was crossing Guerrero Street with her sister in the early evening of February 7, 1950, when she was struck by a car and died instantly. A number of Sisters and personnel witnessed this tragic event. Sister Ambrose was a friend to all at the hospital and is remembered for her great kindness and her ability in the operating room. We had lost another friend three days before her death. On February 4, Bishop James T. O'Dowd, a member of the College of Nursing Advisory Committee and Pastor of our parish church, Mission Dolores, was killed in a car accident.

In 1951, Father Francis Wajda became hospital Chaplain. Father was a seminary professor in his native Poland at the outbreak of World War II. He had spent the war years in four Nazi prison camps—Auschwitz, Birkerau, Flossenburg, and Dachau. Father Wajda was with us twenty-one years, and he influenced all those who came to Mary's Help—patients, visitors, medical staff, employees, Sisters, and students. His priestly zeal and ability to relate and share concerns were extraordinary. Father's letter to all personnel just before his death on April 18, 1972 is expressive of his spirit.

> *Dear Sisters and All Mary's Helpers:*
>
> *So many times did I read the words of our Church Liturgy: "In your mercy keep us free from sin, and protect us from all anxiety as we wait in joyful hope of the coming of Our Lord, Jesus Christ."*

I am now approaching the point where my joyful hope is becoming a vivid, joyful reality.

So many times did I assist the dying in my twenty-one plus years of service at Mary's Help. Every time I stayed with the dying I thought of my own death as surely and inevitably coming to me. I thought of it in terms of our Faith, as some anonymous author presented: "I am standing upon the seashore. A ship at my side spreads her white sails to the morning breeze and starts for the blue ocean. She is an object of beauty and strength and I stand and watch her until at length she hangs like a speck on white cloud just where the sea and sky come down to mingle with each other. Then someone at my side says: 'There she is gone.' Gone where? Gone from my side, that is all. She is just as large in mast and hull as she was when she left my side, and just as able to bear her load of living freight to the place of destination. Her diminished size is in me, not in her. And just at the moment when someone at my side says: 'There she is gone,' there are other eyes watching her coming, and other voices ready to take up the glad shout: 'There she comes.' And that is dying."

I am alone about to join those who "have gone before us marked with the sign of faith," and along with them I will be waiting for all of you, to visit you again one-by-one. Please, do not be less realistic about this than I am.

With all my crowded thoughts in mind, I would like to express my gratitude—

—to the Archbishop and the priests of the Archdiocese of San Francisco, particularly to Bishop Guilfoyle and my Polish fellow-priests for their gift of friendship;

—to all the Sisters, Daughters of Charity—for giving me an opportunity to share in their zeal and dedication in the service of the sick;

—to my personal doctors, to all medical and nursing staff members and to all Mary's Help employees—who have shown me their personal love and deep understanding of my priestly work for the sick;

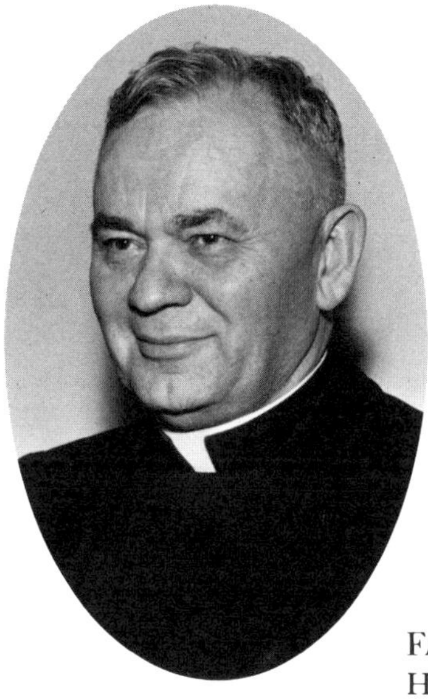

FATHER FRANCIS WAJDA
Hospital Chaplain.

—to all relatives and friends of Mary's Help patients, to all our patients—for their appreciation and generosity given to me for years;

—to all people I came in contact with, to all Polish people in the area—who helped me to take care of their religious needs in the years past.

I ask all and each one of you to forgive many of my shortcomings, and I particularly beg your forgiveness if I ignored, neglected, hurt, or scandalized any one of you.

Thank you, thank you and au revoir, until I see you again.

In the name of the Father, and of the Son, and of the Holy Spirit. Amen.

Francis Wajda

In 1950, Mother Marie Antoinette Blanchot, Superioress General of the Daughters of Charity throughout the world, visited the United States. When she came to Mary's Help, she was welcomed, in French, by Dr. Francis Rochex, President of the Medical Staff, and by Miss Germaine Casabonne (Mrs. Michael Scarfoni), class of 1952, who greeted her on behalf of Mary's Help student nurses.

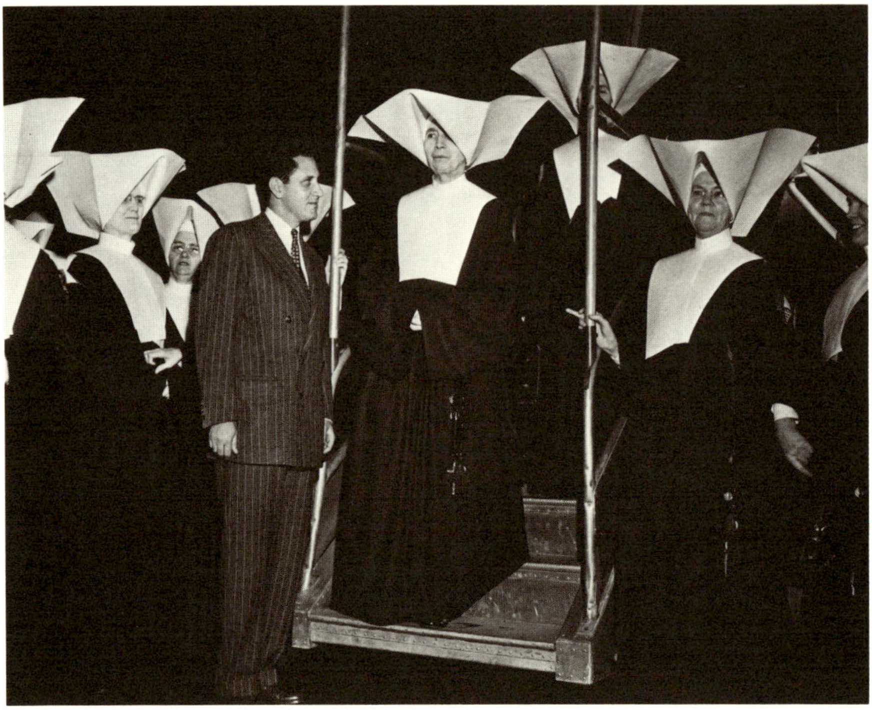

The Most Honored Mother Marie Antoinette Blanchot, Superioress General of the Daughters of Charity, is welcomed to San Francisco in 1950 by local Daughters of Charity and the French Consul.

On September 28, 1952, Archbishop John J. Mitty was the celebrant of the Centennial Mass for the Daughters of Charity in San Francisco at Saint Mary's Cathedral. Students from Mary's Help Hospital were choir members and ushers.

Sister Mary Rose McPhee replaced Sister Alphonsa as Administrator in 1953. The next year Sister established what is now our yearly tradition, the Employee Recognition Dinner. The first service pins were awarded to those who had been employees for twenty years or longer. The top awards were given to Timothy McSweeney, Engineering, 35 years, and Mrs. Grace O'Hanlon, Finance, 29 years. Awards for long-term dedicated service were also given to Edward Garcia, Engineering, and Mrs. Katherine O'Donnell, R.N., Nursing.

Up to this period the hospital operated without a formal public relations program or lay advisory participation such as a board of governors or a community advisory committee. The five-member Board of the Corporation, as stipulated by the will of Mrs. Kate Johnson, was chaired at this time by Archbishop Mitty and met for an annual meeting and special meetings as required.

Sister Mariana Rabe now directed the Clinic services. The growth of the Clinic—over 32,000 patients were seen each year—the range of services provided for the poor, and the substantial costs of nursing

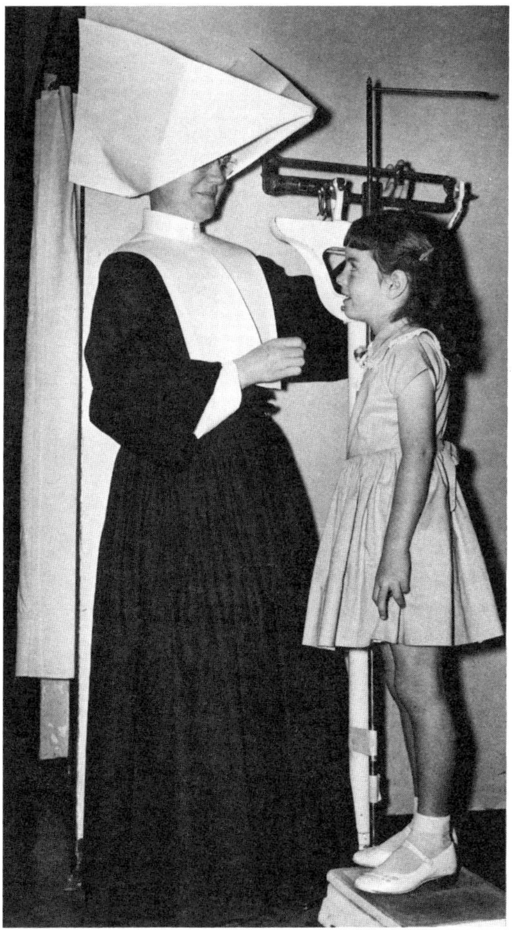

SISTER MARIANA RABE
Working in the Clinic.

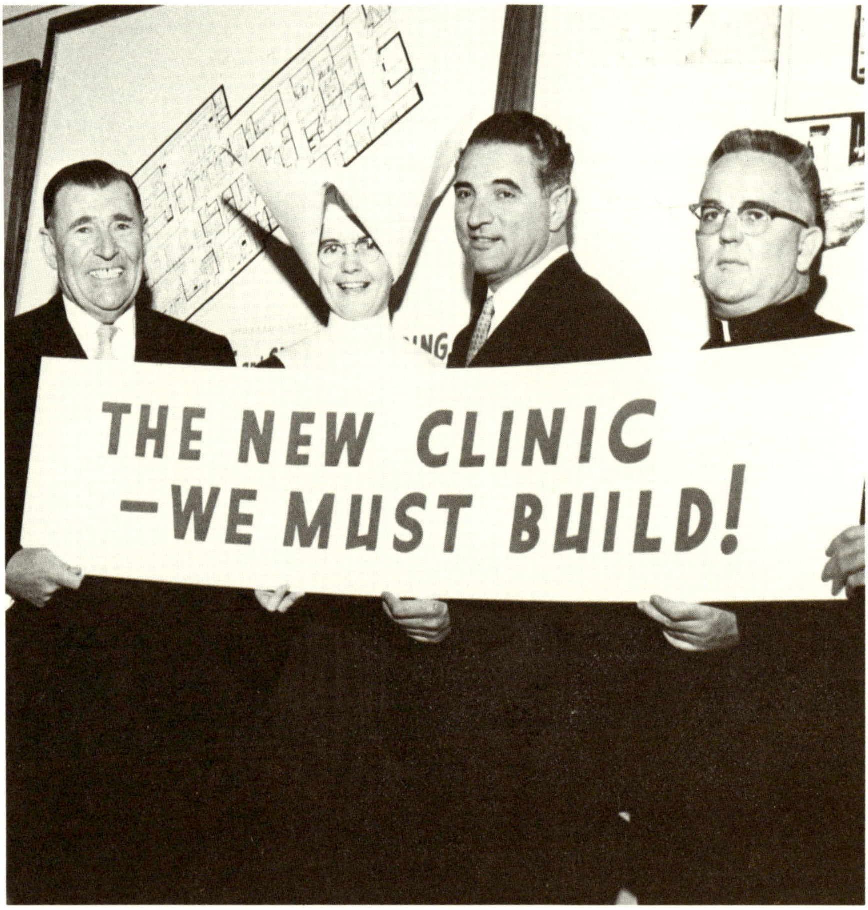

Sister Mary Rose McPhee and fundraisers (l. to r.): Charles Harney, Mayor George Christopher, Msgr. Bernard Cronin.

education made heavy demands on the hospital resources. There was little money to cover depreciation of the old hospital or to fund a new building. By 1954 the advances in medical science and the accompanying growth in the services made our one-and-one-half acre plant hopelessly inadequate. The Clinic, Surgery, and Diagnostic Departments—Radiology, Laboratory, and Physical Therapy—were seriously limited by lack of space. Plans were made to build a million-dollar addition to house a new Surgery Department and Clinic across the street from the hospital.

In 1955, John Lally, Secretary of the Board of Directors of the Corporation from 1929 to 1955, died. Archbishop Mitty appointed James Cummins to the Board. Mr. Cummins served as Secretary and Vice-chairman and remains a valued friend of Mary's Help Hospital and Seton Medical Center.

Jerd F. Sullivan became Chairman of the newly established Fund-Raising Committee in 1956. On April 11, the first public event of the forthcoming drive was held. It was an information luncheon chaired by Charles L. Harney and held at the Palace Hotel. The speakers were:

THE HONORABLE GEORGE CHRISTOPHER,
Mayor of San Francisco
EDDIE JOOST, Manager of the Seals Baseball Club
EDDIE ALBERT, Coach of the Forty-Niners football team
EDGAR V. NOLAN, M.D, member of the
Board of Directors of the Corporation.

Following this event, all the various hospital groups—Medical Staff, Guild, nursing alumnae and friends—began to organize their forces for participation in the public fund drive. Moreover, we had the necessary support of the Board of Supervisors of the City and County of San Francisco. Their resolution of April 15, 1956 commended the work of the Daughters of Charity.

BOARD OF SUPERVISORS
CITY AND COUNTY OF SAN FRANCISCO
Resolution No. 16602

WHEREAS, The Board of Supervisors has noted that Daughters of Charity of St. Vincent de Paul, some 45 years ago opened the first free and low cost clinic under Catholic auspices at Mary's Help Hospital; and

WHEREAS, It is particularly gratifying to the people of San Francisco that the Sisters have continued to work among the sick poor at Mary's Help Clinic under conditions which have been more difficult due to lack of space and facility, and with the aid and services of devoted doctors and hospital staff have under these conditions continued to care for thousands of cases in both their clinic and surgery departments; and

WHEREAS, The Sisters have never appealed to the public for assistance in financing their building program although the fire of 1906 destroyed the hospital plant and the present building has been in use for some 45 years with a continued increase in the number of people cared for; now, therefore, be it

RESOLVED, That the Board of Supervisors of San Francisco does hereby take public cognizance of the contribution that the Daughters of Charity of St. Vincent de Paul—particularly through their work among the poor and needy in Mary's Help Clinic—have made to the health of all the people of San Francisco, and does hereby commend them for their effort to modernize their facilities to better serve the people of our city; and, be it

FURTHER RESOLVED, That a suitably engraved copy of this resolution be tendered to the Daughters of Charity of St. Vincent de Paul at Mary's Help Hospital with the sincere wish that they may enjoy the fullest measure of success and progress in their consecrated work.

I hereby certify that the foregoing resolution was adopted by the Board of Supervisors of the City and County of San Francisco at its meeting of April 16, 1956.

JOHN R. MCGRATH — *Approved, April 18, 1956* — *Clerk*

GEORGE CHRISTOPHER — *April 21, 1956* — *Mayor*

In 1957, the first organized appeal to the people of San Francisco was made on behalf of Mary's Help Hospital. The campaign directors were:

CHRISTIAN DE GUIGNE III, Campaign Chairman

CHARLES L. HARNEY, Chairman of the commercial section of the campaign

DANIEL J. O'HARA, JR., Chairman of the public phase of the campaign

ROBERT A. BILAFER, M.D., Chairman of the Medical Staff; Chairman of the doctors' campaign
ANDREW BURKE, attorney for the Archdiocese
REV. BERNARD J. CRONIN, Archdiocesan Director, Health and Hospitals

The total amount pledged was $320,000.

All plans for rebuilding Mary's Help Hospital were interrupted on Friday, March 22, 1957, at 11:15 a.m. when an earthquake of 5.3 magnitude (the most severe since the 1906 quake) damaged the hospital. Following the earthquake, Sister Mary Rose was notified by the California Department of Health that the plant did not meet the requirements of Article 260 of the Hospital Licensing Act with regard to the hospital's structural condition. At this point, plans for the expansion were tabled. For the next two years the structural condition was studied by consulting engineers and the Board in cooperation with the Bureau of Hospitals, the San Francisco Department of Public Works, and state and city fire officials.

The Board, upon Sister Mary Rose's recommendation, consulted with Sister Basil, former Administrator of the hospital. Sister Basil had done a great deal of remodeling of the plant as well as a tremendous amount of hospital building, particularly in renovating and rehabilitating hospitals throughout the Western Province of the Daughters of Charity. She was known as one of the outstanding "builders" of the Community. Following an intensive review, Sister Basil made the recommendation that it would be unwise to attempt rehabilitation of the present structure for the following reasons:

1. It was impossible to ascertain the cost.
2. Additional requirements were likely to be requested by the San Francisco Fire Commission in the process of the work, if not prior to beginning work.
3. Additional laws would affect the future status of the building and would mean continuous improvement.
4. We would still have an old building which had inadequate facilities.

After many meetings it was decided that the old hospital really could not be rebuilt. A million-dollar refurbishment was not reasonable for a plant built in 1912. It would not be possible to convert the original plant to meet present and future requirements.

Another major problem was our limited space—just one-and-one-half acres. The area in back of the hospital extending to Valencia Street was critical for any expansion on the old site. However, this space was occupied by a factory and a children's playground owned by the Levi Strauss Company. This property was of historical significance and value to them, and they were not willing to sell. Actually, this constraint was a disguised blessing because there was a growing need for hospital facilities in San Mateo County rather than in San Francisco. In a few years Guerrero Street would join the freeway at San Jose Avenue, making the traffic extremely heavy and parking at the Guerrero Street site impossible.

The decision was made to contract with Dr. Anthony J. J. Rourke of New Rochelle, New York, a noted hospital consultant and former Administrator of Stanford Lane Hospital in San Francisco. Dr. Rourke and his associates, notably Miss Louise Esch, conducted an extensive survey. They determined that San Francisco had a surplus of hospital beds while northern San Mateo County had an acute shortage of hospital beds. Daly City had the highest population without hospital and emergency services. The Rourke Report of December 1959 made several final recommendations:

1. The present hospital should be vacated.
2. The beds in Mary's Help Hospital are needed.
3. The Westlake/Daly City area needs hospital and emergency facilities.
4. Mary's Help Hospital, with its long and faithful service in San Francisco, should relocate to a new building and a new location.

Long before Dr. Rourke had been asked to make his survey of health services in the San Francisco area, there was growing concern in northern San Mateo County that hospital services were totally

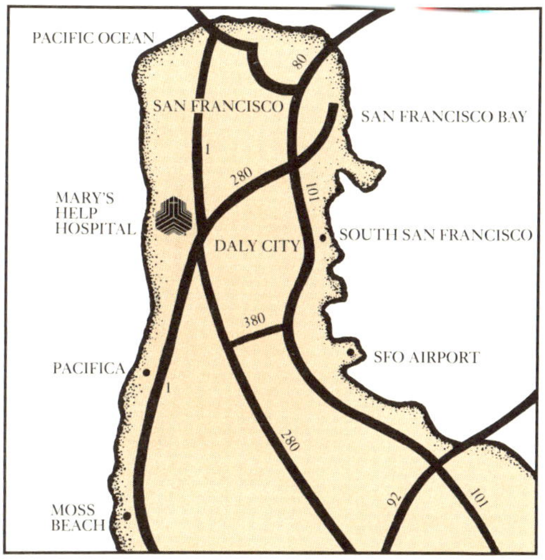

Mary's Help Hospital was located in Northern San Mateo County to serve the San Francisco peninsula, the area found to be in most need of hospital services.

inadequate for the booming population and that continuous high growth necessitated planning hospital services for the future. The mayors of South San Francisco, Daly City, and Pacifica established a Mayors' Hospital Committee to explore ways and means of establishing community hospital services. After careful analysis by the Fact-finding Subcommittee, it was decided that the area should be a hospital service area in the California State Plan for Hospitals. A detailed study was conducted, and a proposal was submitted to the State Advisory Hospital Council. The proposal was approved. The North County area, with a population of 121,000 and the need for 280 general hospital beds, was declared the number one priority area in California.

The College of Nursing continued to thrive during this decade of decisions. In 1955, Mary's Help College of Nursing applied for and received full accreditation from the National League for Nursing. This recognition was granted after an extensive examination of the school's aim and philosophy, curriculum, and educational practices, as well as site visits to both the college and all affiliated educational facilities. The aim and philosophy and the accredited curriculum were as follows.

The Aim and Philosophy of Mary's Help College of Nursing

The aim of the College is to develop and graduate a professional nurse with high principles, capable of promoting the health and general welfare of the community as well as of individuals, and to provide her with a means to attain security and happiness.

At Mary's Help College of Nursing, as in all Catholic education, religion is the integrating factor of the program. Thus the graduate of this program is a better person not only as a result of good training in the art of nursing, but of character training as well.

Our College of Nursing shall in its program of study and practice give evidence that we accept the Catholic concept of the dual nature of man, spiritual and material, joined in substantial union.

We recognize the necessity of developing, to the highest possible degree, those faculties by virtue of which man is human: his reason and his free will.

Because we firmly believe that the end of true education must be wisdom and virtue, our College of Nursing shall endeavor to make possible, through all its activities, such development of the use of right reason and the exercise of free will that our students shall give evidence of wisdom and virtue in their striving toward moral perfection and the attainment of their eternal salvation.

Faith and love of God is the essence of the spirit of St. Vincent, and, therefore, the spirit directing our work.

Curriculum

	Year Taught	*Units*	*Class Hours*	*Clin. Instr.*	*Total Hours*
General Education Courses					
Catholic Philosophy	1		16		16
Philosophy of Life	1		16		16
Moral Philosophy	2		24		24
Philosophy of Values	3		16		16
Biological and Physical Sciences					
Anatomy	1	4	108		108

Physiology	1	4	108		108
Bacteriology	1	4	144		144
Nutrition	1	3	48		48
SOCIAL SCIENCES					
Psychology	1	3	48		48
Sociology	1	3	48		48
INTRODUCTORY NURSING COURSES					
Prof. Relationships I	1		24		24
Prof. Relationships II	3		32		32
Nursing History Trends	1		32		32
Pharmacology I	1		16		16
Nursing I, II	1		198		198
CLINICAL COURSES					
Medical-Surgical Nursing I, II, III	1,2		350	108	458
Orthopedic Nursing	2		16	12	28
Maternal Health Care	2,3		48	36	84
Child Health Care	2,3		48	36	84
Psychiatric Nursing	2,3		76	60	136
Communicable Disease Nursing	2,3		30	29	59
Emergency Nursing and First Aid	3		30	29	59
Problem Solving Seminar	3		22		22
Advanced Medical and Surgical Nursing	3			48	48

CLINICAL EXPERIENCE

	Weeks
Preclinical period	36
Introduction to Medical and Surgical Nursing	4
Medical Nursing	12
Diet Therapy	4
Surgical Nursing and Specialties	8
Surgery	8
Orthopedic Nursing	4
Maternal Health Care	12
Child Health Care	12
Communicable Disease Nursing	4
Psychiatric Nursing	12
Outpatient Department	4
Advanced Medical Nursing	12
Advanced Surgical Nursing	12
Vacation	12
TOTAL	156

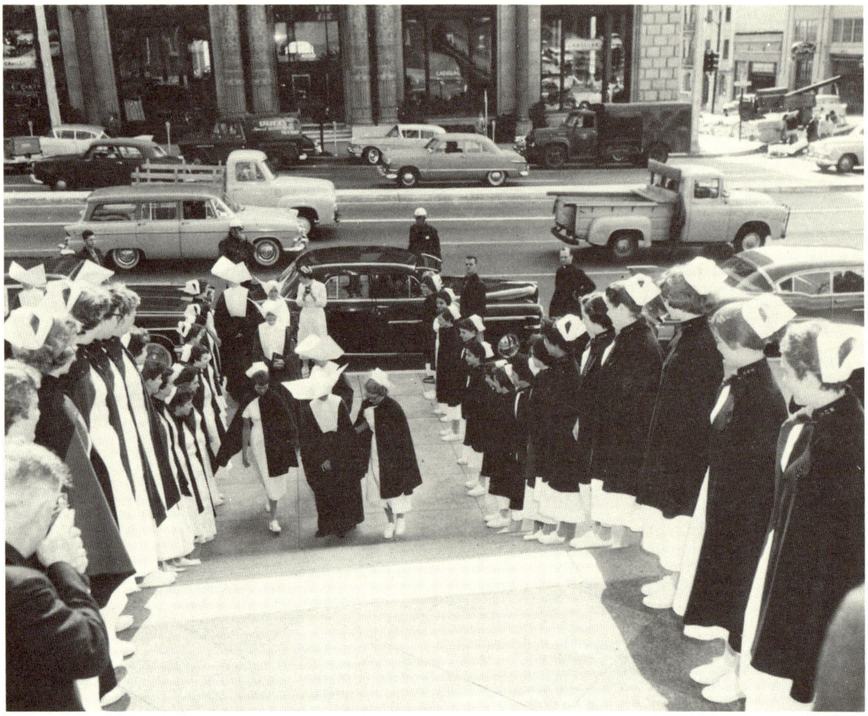

The Most Honored Mother Francine Lepicard, Superioress General of the Daughters of Charity, entering St. Mary's Cathedral on Van Ness Avenue and O'Farrell Street, San Francisco, during her 1958 visit.

This accreditation was the criterion for excellence in nursing education. Receiving it was a reflection of the cooperation between the hospital and the College of Nursing. The students' hours of duty were reduced after accreditation, and more clinical instructors were required. Also as a result of the accreditation, additional nursing service personnel were hired by the hospital.

In this decade, 213 students graduated from the College of Nursing. Sister Ann Leitao was a student nurse in 1953. She left Mary's Help to join the Daughters of Charity in St. Louis. Sister Ann is now Director of Quality Assurance at Seton Medical Center. Sister Eileen Kenny, a former Administrator of the hospital, entered the College of Nursing in 1956. She too left to join the Daughters of Charity. Agnes Malone was an employee at this time (secretary to Sister Mary Rose), and she also left to join the Daughters of Charity in St. Louis. She is now Sister Kevin Malone, Sister Servant at Saint Catherine Hospital On Half Moon Bay. Sister William Eileen Dunn, who at present is a member of our Board of Directors, graduated from the College of Nursing in 1960 and then joined the Daughters of Charity.

On June 8, 1958, Mother Francine Lepicard, Superioress General of the Daughters of Charity, came to San Francisco. She visited Mary's Help Hospital, and a Solemn Mass was offered at Saint Mary's Cathedral on Van Ness Avenue and O'Farrell Streets. Student nurses formed the guard of honor.

In 1959, we established an innovative method of hospital-wide communication called *Operation Daily News*. Every day at ten minutes to four an announcement was made on the hospital's public address system: "Good afternoon. It's ten to four—time for *Operation Daily News*." The announcements were planned as follows:

Monday: Nursing Service Department announcements
Tuesday: Special services announcements—Guild, library, gift shop, volunteers
Wednesday: Safety announcements
Thursday: Safety announcements
Friday: Personnel announcements

Messages from the Administrator and Chaplain were also included. This was a very successful communication device, which was of interest to the entire hospital. *Hospital Progress*, the publication of the Catholic Hospital Association, now Catholic Health Association of the United States, published a report on this service in the December 1959 issue.

During this decade the forces producing change in our system had been in constant motion. Everyone at Mary's Help had exerted extraordinary energy above and beyond the call of duty. Various possibilities for our future had been thoroughly explored; the time for the ultimate decision had arrived.

7

Final Decisions
1960–1965

THE CRITICAL QUESTIONS that had to be answered at this time were: What was to be the fate of the hospital? Could it be rebuilt? Should it move? If so, where? Or should the hospital be closed? What was the future of the College of Nursing? The ramifications of these decisions—in terms of our patients, personnel and the associations of the past fifty years—made the considerations very painful and the decisions, final.

At a special meeting of the Board of the Corporation on January 7, 1960, the following recommendations from Dr. Rourke's study were approved:

1. Discontinue the present plant as soon as it can be replaced.
2. Build a new community general care, short-stay hospital at a site in the general area of Westlake/Daly City.
3. Locate the new hospital on a 15-acre lot to allow for parking and future expansion.

At the same meeting, the time schedule requested by the State Bureau of Hospitals was submitted:

February 1, 1960. Adopt a plan of action based on this report which is acceptable to the Board of the Corporation and the Daughters of Charity. Confer with Mr. Gordon Cumming, Chief of the State Bureau of Hospitals.

February 15, 1960. Secure Archbishop Mitty's approval for a plan of implementation.

March 15, 1960.

1. Secure a site.
2. Appoint an architect and a hospital consultant.
3. Appoint a fund-raising consultant and set dates for a fund campaign.

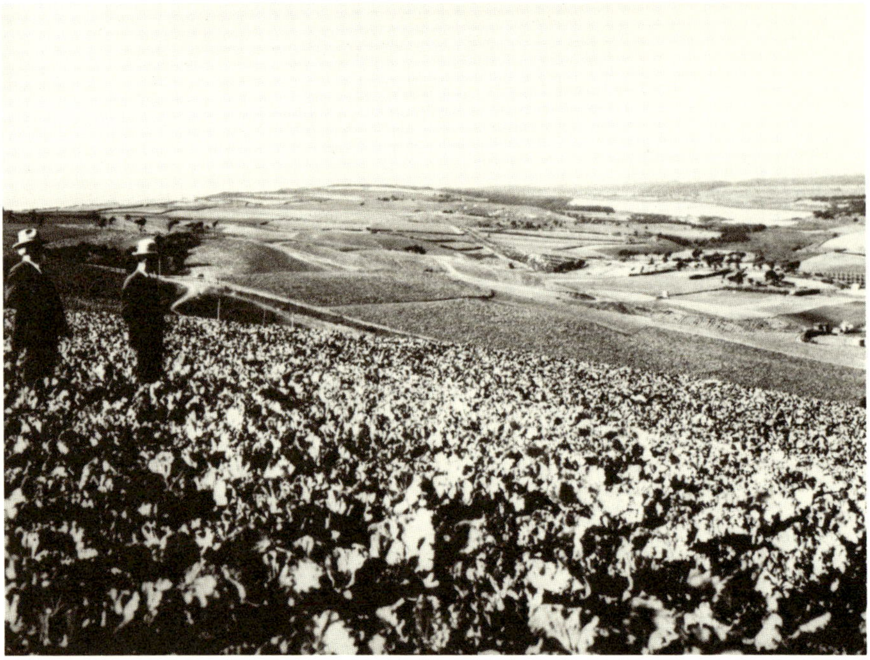

John Daly and James Casey view the Daly City cabbage patch that would become the site of Mary's Help Hospital.

The implementation of the plan became the responsibility of Sister Mary Rose. At the annual meeting of the Board on March 29, 1960, she reported:

1. Gordon Cumming, Chief of the State Bureau of Hospitals, had approved the plans which had been submitted for the necessary work to keep the old hospital operating and for the replacement program.
2. Investigation of suitable available properties was being conducted.
3. Charles Harney was requested to interview a select group of architects and make recommendations.

Sister Hermine Regan replaced Sister Mary Rose as Sister Servant and Administrator in April 1960.

Now that the decision to relocate Mary's Help Hospital was final, the Sisters investigated many possible sites. Due to the generosity of several of our donors, who were developers of the Daly City area, land suitable for a hospital was acquired. In August 1961, the Sisters purchased an eleven-acre area on a hill in Daly City west of Junipero Serra Boulevard in northern San Mateo County. It was convenient to Pacifica, South San Francisco, and twenty-five minutes from downtown San Francisco. The subsequent construction of the freeway, the Serramonte Shopping Center, and the phenomenal growth of the residential area surrounding the site reinforces the wisdom of that choice. The hospital is located at the hub of the transportation routes in northern San Mateo County.

The architectural firm of Stone, Marraccini, and Patterson was selected to plan the project. Dean Folker served as our primary consultant from that firm. Dr. Anthony J. J. Rourke was contracted as consultant for the design and construction of the new hospital. During the time that Lawrence Hoban was Assistant Administrator of Mary's Help, he played a major role in the planning and construction of the new hospital.

Community support and fund-raising were top priorities in May of 1961. George Killion hosted a luncheon for prominent citizens of San Francisco and northern San Mateo County to invite their participation in the construction of the new hospital. A thirty-six member Board of Governors was formed with the Honorable George B. Harris, Chairman, and James Cummins, Vice-chairman. The first committees of the Board of Governors were Finance: Benjamin Swig, Chairman; Public Relations: Eugene Hoffman, Chairman; General Solicitations: Honorable Edward F. O'Day, Chairman.

The Mayors' Hospital Committee, composed of the mayors of Daly City, South San Francisco, and Pacifica, fully supported the hospital since the announcement of the intended move to San Mateo County. Councilman Leo J. Ryan of South San Francisco, chairman of the Fact-finding Subcommittee, Frank Pacelli of Daly City and Harold Feyge of Pacifica were particularly active in hospital affairs. This subcommittee worked successfully on the proposal for the creation of a new hospital service area under the Hill-Burton program and also obtained City Council action in support of Mary's Help Hospital's move to the Daly City area. Various chambers of commerce and medical groups also endorsed Mary's Help Hospital's plans.

In October 1961, Mary's Help Hospital received a Hill-Burton grant of $3,800,000 to build a new 250-bed hospital. On March 19, 1962, His Excellency, Joseph T. McGucken became Archbishop of San Francisco and assumed the position of President of the Board of Directors of the Corporation replacing Archbishop John J. Mitty.

In 1962, the fifty-year agreement between the Daughters of Charity and the Corporation for the Daughters to conduct Mary's Help Hospital expired. A resolution was adopted by the Corporation authorizing the Daughters of Charity to conduct and manage the hospital and to enter into contracts.

On April 5, 1963, the Corporation was transferred to the Community of the Daughters of Charity by Archbishop McGucken, President of the Corporation. At that time, the members of the Board of the Corporation resigned. They were Archbishop Joseph T. McGucken,

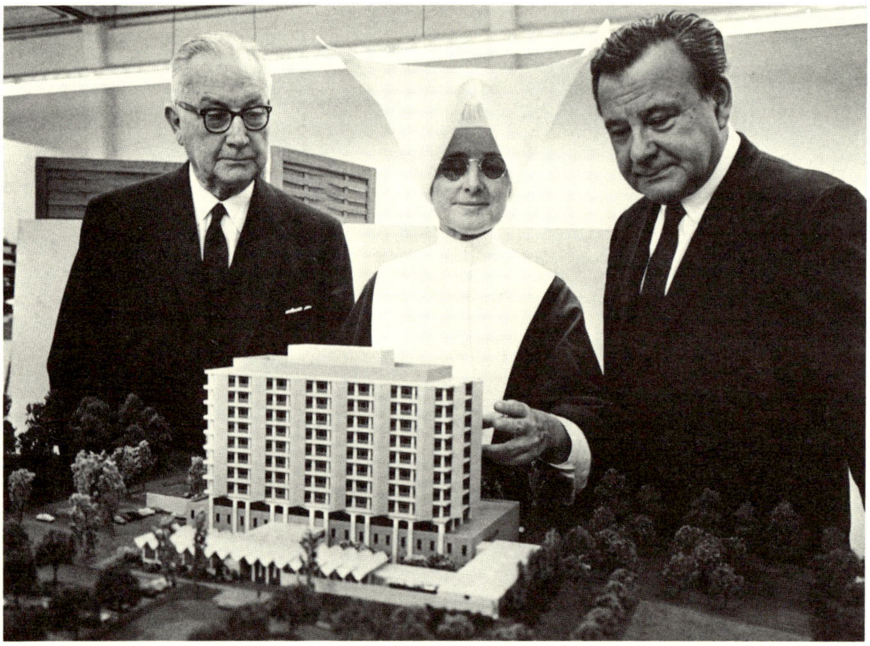

Roy Bronson, Sister Hermine Regan and Judge George Harris look at a model of the new hospital to be constructed in Daly City.

President; James Cummins, Vice-president; Robert A. Bilafer, M.D., member; Edgar V. Nolan, M.D., member.

Corporate control passed from the lay Board to the Daughters of Charity. The newly appointed Board members were Sister Hermine Regan, President; Sister Benedicta Burkhart, Secretary-Treasurer; Sister Mary Thomas Redd, Vice-president; Sister Sebastian Casey, member; and Sister Dorothy Bachelot, member.

At the same meeting on April 5, 1963, the following resolutions passed.

Resolution Commending the Daughters of Charity of St. Vincent de Paul

> Dr. Bilafer moved that the Board of Directors express their appreciation for the generosity and selfless work of the Daughters of Charity of St. Vincent de Paul at Mary's Help Hospital, for their efficiency in the conduct of the hospital operation, and for their devotion to the humanitarian work of aiding the sick for the love and honor of God. Dr. Bilafer further moved that the Board go on record as expressing its willingness, both collectively and individually, to continue to work with and for the Sisters in the future. The motions were seconded by Dr. Nolan and carried unanimously.

Sister Hermine read the following Resolution which had been unanimously adopted by the Daughters of Charity at Mary's Help Hospital:

Resolution of Appreciation from the Daughters of Charity

> *WHEREAS*, His Excellency, the Most Reverend Archbishop of San Francisco, and his predecessors, together with a select group of contemporary members of the clergy and laity, have served respectively as President and Chairman of the Board, and Board Members of Mary's Help Hospital Corporation for more than half a century, and,
>
> *WHEREAS*, these distinguished prelates and their contemporary fellow officers and board members through-

> out the years gave unstintingly of their time, energy and substance in the best interest of Mary's Help Hospital, and,
>
> *WHEREAS*, by virtue of their selfless dedication, wise counsel and always loyal devotion to the duties and responsibilities of their respective offices, they have created an institution that is more than a mere hospital—an institution which, by the Grace of God and Mary's help has succeeded in living, quietly and unsung, the spirit and letter of God's second Great Commandment: 'Love thy neighbor as thyself.' Be it therefore
>
> *RESOLVED*, that the Daughters of Charity of St. Vincent de Paul do hereby recognize and acknowledge, with deep humility and prayerful thanks, their great debt of gratitude to the Most Reverend Joseph T. McGucken, Archbishop of San Francisco, and his predecessors, and to the retiring officers and board members of Mary's Help Hospital Corporation: Mr. James Cummins, Dr. Robert A. Bilafer and Dr. Edgar V. Nolan, and be it further
>
> *RESOLVED*, that these, and all other benefactors of Mary's Help Hospital—many of whom have already been called to their reward—will always be gratefully and devoutly remembered in our prayers.

On behalf of the Daughters of Charity, Sister Hermine expressed appreciation and gratitude for the direction and assistance given to Mary's Help Hospital during the past few years by the Reverend Timothy E. O'Brien, Director of Health and Hospitals for the Archdiocese of San Francisco.

Mayor Joseph Verducci welcomed us to Daly City at the public ground-breaking ceremonies on May 11, 1963. Archbishop Joseph McGucken was the principal speaker. Presiding was Judge George B. Harris, the dedicated leader of the fund-raising efforts for the new hospital. Construction began on the following day.

The status and future of our College of Nursing was an agonizing concern during this period. From the time the first students entered in

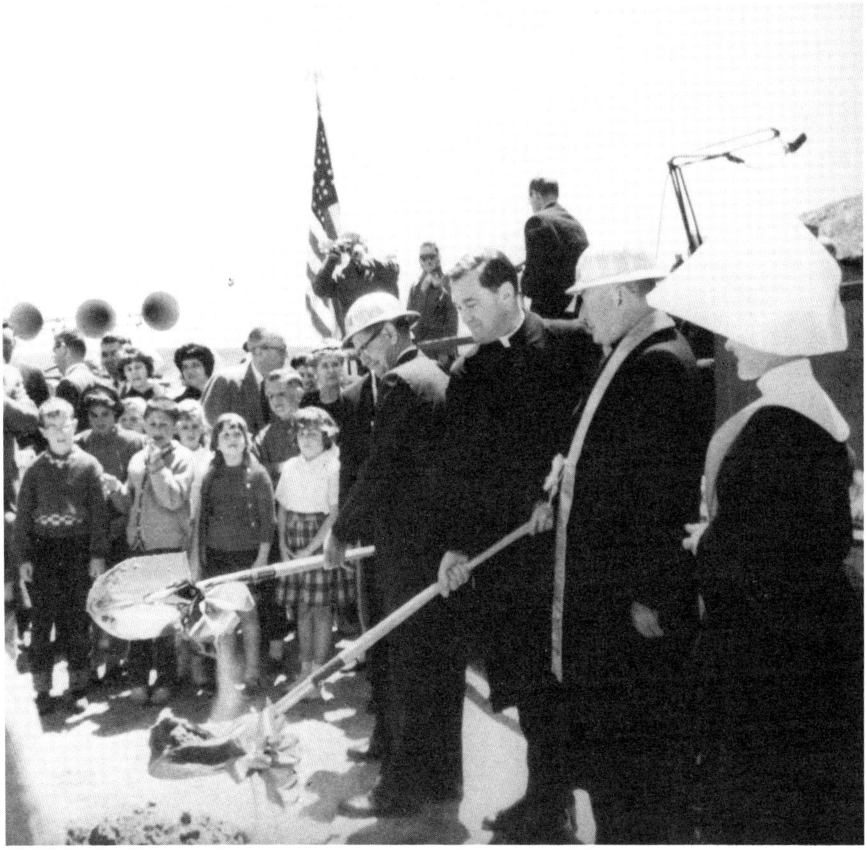

Ground-breaking ceremonies in May 1963 for the new Mary's Help Hospital in Daly City. Reverend Timothy O'Brien, Director of Health and Hospitals for the Archdiocese of San Francisco; Archbishop Joseph McGucken; and Sister Hermine Regan.

1912, the college had always been an integral part of the hospital. The program, which was one of the first to receive state accreditation and which received accreditation from the National League of Nursing in 1955, was regarded as excellent. The students were a source of pride and satisfaction to the Sisters, to the medical staff, and to the entire hospital.

Nevertheless, it was decided that the College of Nursing would be closed. Some reasons for the closing were our relocation, changes in nursing education including the trend in California to place nursing education in a collegiate setting, and the spiraling cost of maintaining an accredited hospital program. Although the nursing students would be missed by patients and staff alike, there was the conviction that the decision was appropriate. It was our Director of Nursing, Jessie Miller, who came to Mary's Help Hospital in 1953, who had the difficult assignment of closing the school in 1963. Some of the key individuals who had supplied the leadership for the nursing education program from 1912 to 1963 were Sister Martha Lawlor, Sister Dolores Carlos, Sister Stephanie Wall, Sister Eligius Chesbro, Sister Dorothea Bertoneau, Sister Virginia Boos, Sister Clare Neuhoff, and Miss Jessie Miller.

Members of the last class to graduate, in 1963, were:

Carol Baker
Linda Banks
Gladys Beierschmitt
Sandra Bianco
Carrie Boegle
Pennie Broadfoot
Theresa Cerizo
Patricia Comphel
Sharon Engstrom
Sandra Figoni
Judy Hamlet
Rita Jones
Ann Micheletti
Ann Panagakis
Silvina Ramirez
Patricia Ricci
Joyce Rodriguez
Barbara Salac
Adele Silva
Rita Walker
Elizabeth Wright
Judith Wyrsch
Jenalee Wheeler

The varied problems associated with closing the College of Nursing were painful to many. It was not easy to observe the passing of an excellent institution of nursing education. It was difficult to see people displaced and the nurses' residences dismantled.

The one happy outcome involved our College of Nursing dog, Linus. We had had him for years. He was a stray of undetermined origin and tremendous personality who came to us and became our mascot. When the College of Nursing closed, Linus retired to Carmel with Mrs. Ellen Reynolds, our housemother.

8

The Move
December 12, 1965

THE TASK OF MOVING A HOSPITAL is always a major project, and moving Mary's Help Hospital from Guerrero Street in San Francisco to Sullivan Avenue in Daly City was indeed a challenge. Mary's Help was a hospital in the City and County of San Francisco, and now would become a community hospital in San Mateo County. It had grown from a small facility to a large one within a newly created hospital district.

The move represented change for everyone involved, but detailed planning facilitated adjustment to the change. The dream of a new hospital made the changes easier for us. The uncertainties were over. Answers to the questions of what *was* and *would be* Mary's Help Hospital were clear. We had a new beginning—high on a hilltop in Daly City.

On Sunday, December 12, 1965, at 10:05 a.m., an announcement was made by the new Administrator, Sister Louise Scheessele, who had replaced Sister Hermine in 1964.

> *Mary's Help Hospital*
> *145 Guerrero Street*
> *San Francisco, California 94103*
> *Underhill-3-0733*
>
> *is now*
>
> *Mary's Help Hospital*
> *1900 Sullivan Avenue*
> *Daly City, California 94015*
> *992-4000*
>
> *The move is completed. Our patients have arrived safely and are now resting in their rooms.*

The announcement made the move seem simple, but in reality it reflected years of planning and decisions, and months of intense preparation and work.

In January 1964, plans for the new *Administrative Policy Manual* were finalized. This book was a source document for planning the move. The manual was significant to our move because it helped us to recognize that one of the more successful methods of coping with change is meaningful communication. It served as a reference for policies, systems and standards, and, superimposed upon these, our procedures. This documentation helped us standardize and formalize our policies and enabled us to perform new activities and make sound decisions expeditiously. A portion of the policy manual that was critical to the success of the move was the section on interdepartmental relations. We would have many departments in the new hospital that did not exist in the old one—for example, Respiratory Therapy. To ensure uniformity of operations, department managers outlined their procedures in the new facility using a standard format.

A great amount of time was spent by upper level management and department managers in developing departmental philosophies that were based on the Philosophy Statement of the Health Care Apostolate of the Daughters of Charity. This statement of basic beliefs directs our actions at every level of the organization. The section in the manual on interdepartmental relations was tremendously valuable because it spelled out the relationships between departments and showed us that we were all working toward the same goal—that is, quality patient care and service.

As the time for the move drew closer, we were increasingly pressured to complete such tools as the orientation outlines, departmental procedure books, staffing patterns, operation plans for new systems, and directions for the move. Our excitement grew. In late September 1965, a schedule was distributed to all department managers with the directive that they would prepare an outline showing how they would plan and execute the move while maintaining services at the old hospital.

Schedule of the Move
October—December 1965

MONDAY October 11, 1965	Delivery of equipment begins, continuing through December 1, 1965.
MONDAY October 18	Purchasing department opened in Daly City. Set up of patient room furniture on floors 7 down thru 3 commenced.
THURSDAY November 4 & FRIDAY November 5	Final check-out of systems.
MONDAY November 8	Department managers tours at 1:30 p.m.
WEDNESDAY November 10	Final inspection by Bureau of Hospitals (H.B. and Licensing Divisions), USPHS, State Fire Marshal, City of Daly City.
THURSDAY November 11 & FRIDAY November 12	Employee tours.
FRIDAY November 12	Press conference and tour at 1:30 p.m.
MONDAY November 15	Acceptance from contractor; filing of Notice of Completion; owner assumes responsibility for building. Opening of library and transfer of inventory. Issue of keys to department managers and assumption by department managers of responsibility for cleaning and setting up departments (individual department time tables to be established prior to this day); intensive orientation and training of personnel to commence. Transfer of furniture "on hand" to commence. Special preview tours to commence with tour by City Council of Daly City; tours thru December 1.

MONDAY November 22	Close fourth medical floor (19 beds) and transfer personnel to new hospital. Delivery of supplies (except perishables and pharmacy) to old Mary's Help to stop. Delivery of supplies to new hospital to start.
WEDNESDAY November 24	Special tour for Medical/Dental staff 1-3 p.m.
TUESDAY November 30	Laundry to open (with truck service to old Mary's Help). Partial opening of Central Supply.
THURSDAY December 2	State and federal inventory of equipment.
FRIDAY SATURDAY SUNDAY December 3, 4, 5	Open house; conducted tours 10 a.m. to 12 noon; 2-4 p.m. (Ground, 5, 6, 7th floors excluded).
MONDAY December 6	Open cafeteria (10 a.m.—4 p.m.); limited service.
TUESDAY December 7	Close O.R. in old Mary's Help except for emergency surgery. Close Clinic in old Mary's Help (no clinic from Dec. 7 to 12, inclusive).
WEDNESDAY December 8	Close first medical floor (16 beds). Medical/Dental staff, active staff meeting, 6:30 p.m. (Classroom). Medical/Dental staff dinner 7:30 p.m. (Cafeteria).
THURSDAY & FRIDAY December 9, 10	Close surgical patient units, one at a time, when possible.
FRIDAY December 10	4 p.m., discontinue admissions to Obstetrical Department (arrangements with St. Mary's for Clinic patients between 4 p.m. Friday and 12 noon Sunday, December 12).
SUNDAY December 12	Opening of hospital in Daly City including Emergency Department. Transfer of patients from old Mary's Help.

MONDAY December 13	Opening of clinic in Emergency Department.
THURSDAY December 16	Open house for employees, alumnae, auxiliary, Medical/Dental staff members.
SATURDAY December 18	Dedication 3 p.m.
	Civic reception dinner hosted by the City of Daly City 6:30 p.m.
SUNDAY December 19	Dedication Mass, hospital chapel 10:00 a.m.

The Department of Education used the moving schedule as a guide in organizing a hospital-wide education program. The content of the education program was organized on three levels: first, a series of programs on change—the process, reactions, and facilitators; second, programs on philosophy and general policies, and classes on hospital emergencies, fire alarm systems, and disaster; and third, specific orientation and teaching outlines for each hospital department.

The education process for the move to the new facility had a unique beginning. Early in 1965 we started the process with hospital-wide classes on the fire alarm system and fire safety practices in the new building. Because the new hospital was the first high-rise building in the area we were requested by the Daly City Fire Department to include their members in these classes. The firemen came as students to our first class in the old hospital. Later they continued with classes in the new building. Actually, this marked the beginning of a very cooperative relationship between Mary's Help and the Daly City Fire Department. They have always been actively involved and interested in our fire safety.

The thoroughness of our planning extended to Mary's Help Hospital Ladies of Charity and their projects. Their contributions to the sick poor were in the tradition of the works of St. Vincent de Paul and St. Louise de Marillac. St. Vincent recognized that to serve the sick poor effectively, there should be two types of helpers. The Daughters of Charity serve as the working group, while the Ladies of Charity supply the necessary resources and assistance. As early as the Fall of 1913, there was a group of women at Mary's Help Hospital that was devoted to supplying material aid to our Clinic patients and other needy families. The names of all the women who contributed to this cause are too numerous to list in this account.

At the time of the move, Mrs. Julia Golden, wife of Dr. John Golden, led the Ladies of Charity. She had reorganized the group in 1958 and provided leadership until her death in June 1968. Mrs. Golden was very devoted to the poor and motivated the Mary's Help Hospital Guild and hospital staff to supply the needy with food and clothing on a regular basis. Our first Christmas party for the Clinic children was in 1913, and this practice was continued each year. At a November 1965 department managers meeting, Mrs. Golden announced that the Clinic Christmas party and Christmas baskets for the needy had been taken care of at Thanksgiving this year. Realizing that

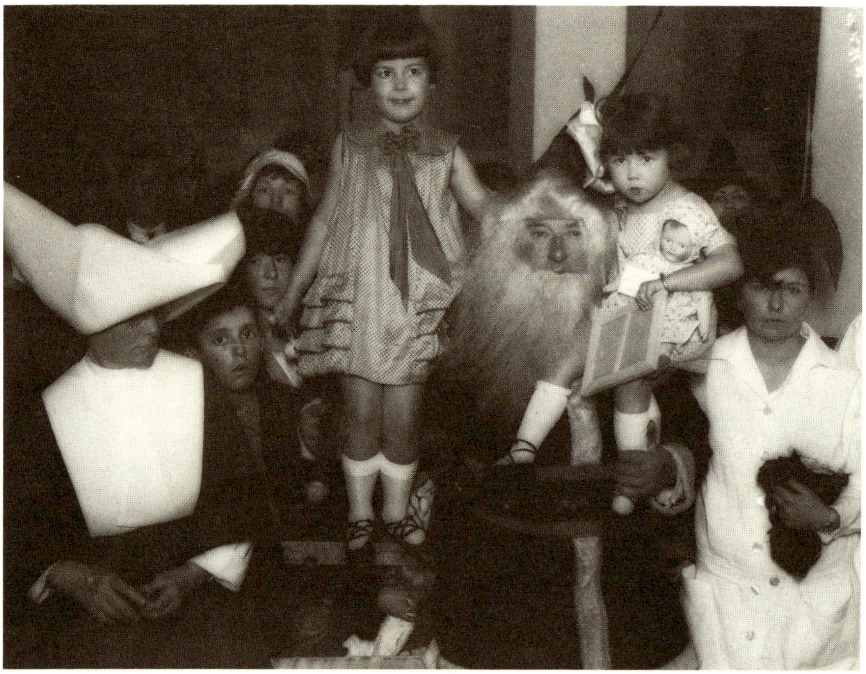

Sister Agatha Flynn and a group of children greet Santa at an early annual Clinic Christmas party at Mary's Help Hospital, San Francisco.

we would be in Daly City in December, she had scheduled two sets of Christmas activities: one for San Francisco Clinic patients in November and a second round in Daly City immediately after the move. Once we were settled, Mrs. Golden reorganized her group and began the same projects here.

While we were working to complete our moving plans, the Daly City officials made every effort to assist us and to make us feel welcome. Frank Pacelli, Mayor of Daly City at that time, was a very strong supporter of our interests. He was one of the several individuals who helped us to obtain the site, change the hospital district boundaries to gain eligibility for Hill-Burton funds, and sponsor our fund drive. These are just some of the projects that our friends in Daly City, South San Francisco, and Pacifica worked on for the new Mary's Help Hospital. Another such friend was Monsignor Richard W. Power, Pastor of Our Lady of Mercy Church in Daly City. He was a member of the Lay Advisory Board and an enthusiastic advocate of the new hospital. He was able to mobilize the manpower for the fund drive in Daly City.

The following official statement issued by Mayor Frank Pacelli of Daly City on behalf of the City Council and city administration is expressive of their support.

> *We welcome the Daughters of Charity and Mary's Help Hospital to the Daly City community. In addition, we recognize that this wonderful facility will be immediately available to residents of Pacifica, San Bruno, South San Francisco and other parts of northern San Mateo County as well as to Daly City and San Francisco.*
>
> *It will be the newest and most modern hospital on the Peninsula and the people of this community are proud to have been able to participate and to have been a factor in locating this new hospital in our area.*
>
> *The hospital will not only enhance the area with its imposing edifice, but will also be an important factor in our community life, generating business sales, the construction of other new buildings, and an increase in population. In general, it will stimulate the economy of the surrounding area. It will also provide for a complete and very sorely needed emergency hospital service.*

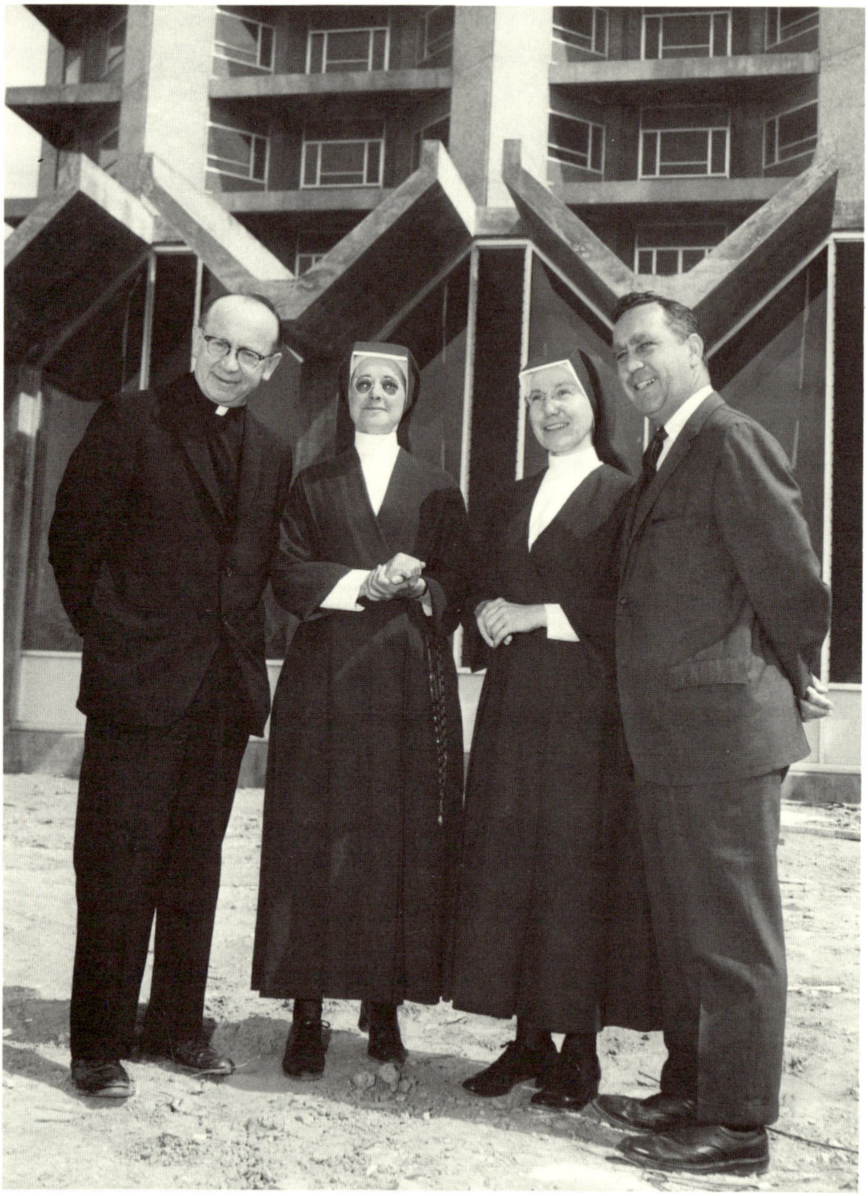

Msgr. Richard Power and Mayor Francis Pacelli welcome Mary's Help Hospital to Daly City; shown here with Sister Hermine Regan and Sister Louise Scheessele.

Possibly the most gratifying aspect of this new hospital service is that in this day of spiraling taxes and bond issues, it is wonderful to have a hospital of this size come into our community and be self-supporting. We have acquired an $8.5 million enterprise without the tax-payers of Daly City or the surrounding areas being taxed for a modern hospital.

We are looking forward to a continued fine relationship with the Daughters of Charity, the Mary's Help Hospital Administration and all those who were a part of the efforts in making this the outstanding project of this year for Daly City.

Preparing for the move was exciting for all of us. It was really fun for the hospital employees to drive in caravans of cars from Guerrero Street to Daly City. Actually, we were lost many times because the freeways had not been built, and it was not always easy to find the new hospital or the right road to the new hospital.

We spent many hours at the new facility having classes, demonstrating new systems, and planning for the placement of all the equipment and supplies so that there would be uniformity throughout the entire nursing tower. We also spent a great deal of time completing the work on the departmental procedure books.

Extensive tours of the new hospital were carefully planned. While the crowds of people who came to see the facility were very welcome, the numbers were unexpected. We had not anticipated that the new hospital would generate such tremendous interest in the Daly City community.

Our time-tested communication device, *Operation Daily News*, assumed a new function during the move. In addition to making announcements on the audio-page, we established a written publication to supply information regarding new equipment, coming events, functions and responsibilities. The first printed issue of *Operation Daily News* was distributed on November 26, 1965. This publication was the forerunner of the Department of Education's current publication, *Education News & Notes*. Since its origin in 1965, this publication has never failed to meet a deadline!

A few issues of *Operation Daily News* and two announcements from Sister Louise offer firsthand accounts of the move and its impact on us.

FIRST ISSUE

Operation Daily News

Friday, November 26, 1965 — *Issue No. 1*

Here we are with a new format—*Operation Daily News* has come to life. Do you remember it as a series of announcements on the audio-page every afternoon at 10 to 4? Well, here it is in print—a special supplement on the move to Daly City.

Someone should record for posterity the events of the move, and lacking a Boswell, we will have to do it ourselves.

Have you noticed the "new" look at the "old" Mary's Help: mismatched chairs and tables, administrative desks replaced by tables and other odd pieces? People carrying boxes with a rather furtive look as they prepare for the move? Mrs. Ellen Reynolds is seen all over the hospital casting her knowing eyes over our remaining furniture, marking it, and then the next day, it's gone. Then, there are the people with the planning jobs that are never seen without sheets and folders. Each time you look down the main corridor, there are little groups of employees with coats, scarfs, and often umbrellas, and perhaps packages, going out to the new hospital, and there are other groups returning. Everyone greets everyone else with a question, "How about this?" "How are we going to do that?" "Have you thought about this?" The tempo has changed and the tempers, too, but let's look upon the move as the great adventure—it really is.

On Monday, November 22nd, the interdepartmental meeting was held at the new hospital. Sister Louise and Mr. Hoban brought us up to date on the move.

The program for teaching for the new hospital was given to the department managers and they will be responsible for seeing that everyone will have an opportunity—well let's face it, it's a command performance—to attend the demonstration of the equipment for the new hospital.

You know from your tours that there is much to learn and we all have to know how to use the new phone system, the pneumatic tubes, the trayvayors, etc. Keep watching for announcements. Keep asking your department managers if there are any scheduled demonstrations. Remember, learning about the new hospital is everyone's business.

Demonstrations now Scheduled are:

1. Trayvayor and Pneumatic Tubes	2:00 p.m. Monday, Nov. 29
2. Trayvayor and Pneumatic Tubes	2:00 p.m. Tuesday, Nov. 30
3. Trayvayor and Pneumatic Tubes	2:00 p.m. Wednesday, Dec. 1
4. Telephone System	10:00 a.m. & continue thru day, Thursday, Dec. 2
5. Nurse's Call & Intercom's	2:00 p.m. Thursday, Dec. 2
6. Nurse's Call & Intercom's	2:00 p.m. Friday, Dec. 3

Assemble for these at the loading dock of the New Hospital.

Watch, too, for the next edition of *Operation Daily News*. Things are going so fast you can't afford to miss anything.

LETTER FROM FATHER WAJDA

Operation Daily News

Friday, December 10, 1965 *Issue No. 8*

Special Issue From Reverend Francis Wajda, Hospital Chaplain:

We are about to move our patients and God's most loved darlings from the old to the new Mary's Help Hospital. But before the ambulances start running, Sunday, December 12, 1965, we are prayerfully mindful of his words: "Without me, you can do nothing." We will escort Him to the exit door of the old and greet Him at the entrance door of the new Mary's Help Hospital with the warm: "Come Lord Jesus and stay with and amidst us."

To make this religious experience meaningful to our patients and to ourselves, the following proceedings will be observed:

> Fifteen minutes before the departure of the first ambulance (7:45 A.M.), Our Lord, carried by the Chaplain, will be escorted by the Sisters and the present personnel to the ambulance entrance door. There, they kneel in adoration until the Chaplain departs.
>
> The receiving station at the new Mary's Help Hospital will be notified that the moving proceedings have started and that the arrival of the Blessed Sacrament is expected in approximately twenty minutes.
>
> At the receiving station (Emergency Entrance), personnel and Sisters will be waiting. As soon as the Chaplain leaves the car, all present will kneel in adoration until two Sisters with candles escort Our Lord to our temporary chapel.

Letter From Sister Louise to Patients Transferred From Old Hospital and To All Patients Admitted, December 12, 1965

MARY'S HELP HOSPITAL
1900 Sullivan Avenue
Daly City, California

December 12, 1965

Dear ______________________

You are our long-anticipated guest. To you, one of our first patients in the new hospital, we extend a very warm welcome!

The only reason for the new building, the equipment and all of this large facility, is you. Our only concern is your welfare and providing you with the finest medical and nursing care possible.

In the name of the Sisters, the medical-dental staff and the personnel, we welcome you to Mary's Help Hospital and ask God's blessing upon you and your loved ones.

Sister Louise
Hospital Administrator

MOVING DAY ISSUE

Operation Daily News

Sunday, December 12, 1965 *Issue No. 9*

M-DAY – MOVE – MEMORIES – MIRROR OF THE FUTURE

The momentous day, Dec. 12, 1965, long anticipated, is here! All of the projects, preparations, and plans are being tested today when the new Mary's Help Hospital goes into operation.

Administration and personnel are all keyed to the change, and from our cooperative efforts we hope will emerge an effective team for the transfer of operations from the old to the new.

We hope, too, that all that was the very best in us in the old hospital, will be magnified here in the new hospital.

Now for some specific directions:

1. On Sunday, during the move, all personnel are expected to remain in their own area. To effect the transfer of patients smoothly and efficiently, all personnel are needed at their assigned stations. *Please remain there.*

2. This beautiful new building is a delight to all of us, but it is also a challenge. To maintain the property as it is now, we have to be careful as we use the equipment, the building, the furniture, all of it. It is all new and beautiful; it is Mary's Help; let's keep it as it is.

3. Keep in mind our directives for the use of equipment. In the paramedical office we have some extra copies of *Operation Daily News* so you can complete your set of instructions.

4. The new facility also calls for a new look in personnel. Our grooming should match the building. Let's reflect in our appearance the style and beauty of the hospital.

5. A final note today is the hospital code for cardiac arrest. It is Code 99. When you hear "Code 99, room _____," this is notification that there is a cardiac arrest emergency. For specific directions and complete information, see the administrative policy book, part V, pages 43 to 48.

Sister Louise's Letter of Thanks to all Personnel

December 13, 1965

TO EACH AND EVERYONE OF YOU:

A Promise Made Is Like A Debt Unpaid

To everyone associated with the move from the old to the new Mary's Help, we have made a mental note to express personally what we feel, our most sincere thanks. But since it is not possible to speak with each of you today, please accept this note as an expression of our sincere and heartfelt gratitude.

The task and the planning, the building, the period of construction, maintaining the old hospital, and finally the move to the new, was a tremendous one, but you were more than equal to the challenge and, due to your efforts, the move took place with magnificent organization and efficiency.

Groups assisting in the patient transfer, the various ambulance companies, the office of civil defense, also expressed their admiration for the way everything was planned and the smoothness and rapidity of this operation. Everyone noticed also, that the dominant theme in the move was "universal concern" for the welfare of our patients.

Throughout all the past preparation and planning, your constant awareness of patient needs and your demands that everything be centered about the patient, was an inspiration and a challenge to us. Be assured that we are both aware and impressed with the spirit which has characterized the "Old Mary's Help" and will strive with you to maintain and magnify it in the "New Mary's Help."

You have expended both your time and talents most generously and we are truly thankful. It is our sincere wish that you and your loved ones will enjoy a Holy and a Happy Christmas, and we invite you to participate in our "CHRISTMAS OPEN HOUSE" on Thursday, December 23rd, from 8 a.m. to 4 p.m.

Sister Louise
Hospital Administrator

On December 12, all the people working in the old hospital were on duty very early to get ready for the transfer, which had been planned and rehearsed the previous week. There were twenty-seven patients to be transferred, and twenty-seven ambulances, donated by all the local ambulance services, were waiting for them. Each patient had a pre-assigned nurse and a volunteer for the transfer. Family members were also invited to ride in the ambulance if they wished. Patient records were completed according to a standard format. Each ambulance was dispatched from the ambulance entrance on Clinton Park in San Francisco. It was accompanied by representatives of the San Francisco Civil Defense Disaster Council and Corps, who were of tremendous assistance during the move. Special thanks go to William Conroy, who was in charge of the Corps, and Louis Cambou, an old friend of ours who was working with the Disaster Council.

Our caravan of ambulances followed Mission Street to Daly City

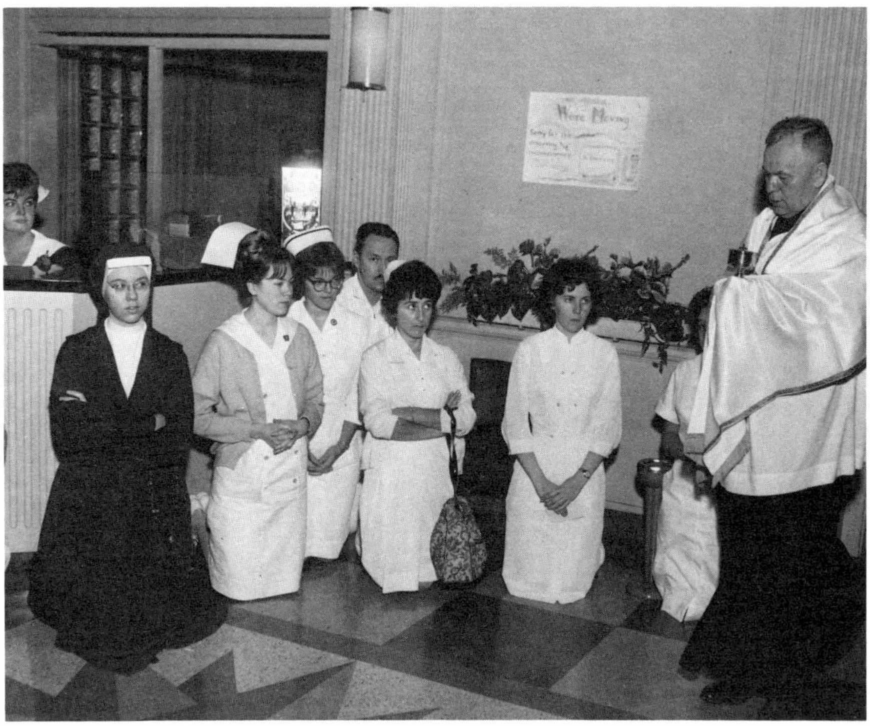

Father Francis Wajda transfers the Blessed Sacrament from the old hospital, Sunday, December 12, 1965.

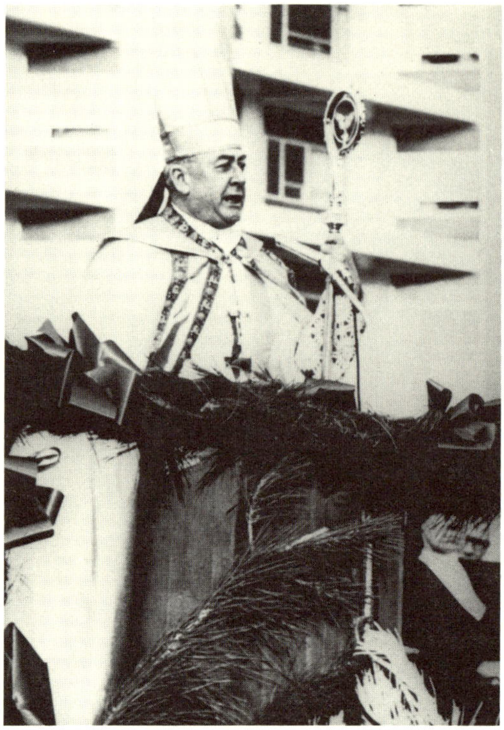

ARCHBISHOP JOSEPH MCGUCKEN
Dedicating Mary's Help Hospital in Daly City, on Saturday, December 18, 1965.

and up the hill to the hospital. Sister Louise, the Administrator, and a group of physicians received the patients when they arrived at the Emergency entrance of the new hospital. The patients were immediately dispatched to their pre-assigned rooms. Guild members and nurses were available to escort patients to the rooms. By 10:00 in the morning the entire cortege of patients had been transferred from San Francisco to Daly City.

The Emergency Department began to function immediately. The people of Daly City welcomed an Emergency facility so heartily that this service was busy from the first day. One of our first patients at the new hospital was a woman who delivered twins shortly before noon on Sunday, December 12. As the week progressed, more and more patients were admitted.

Both old and new staff shared the interest and excitement in anticipation of the upcoming dedication ceremony on Saturday,

Dedication Program

3 p.m. Saturday, December 18, 1965 *Mary's Help Hospital*

Monsignor Richard W. Power, Master of Ceremonies

INVOCATION.. Rev. Thomas J. Farrell

NATIONAL ANTHEM.................................... Jefferson High School Band, Daly City

PLEDGE OF ALLEGIANCE .... Daly City Chorus

INTRODUCTION OF PLATFORM GUESTS............... Msgr. Richard W. Power

Greetings

The Honorable Francis Pacelli, Mayor of Daly City

The Honorable John F. Shelley, Mayor of San Francisco

His Excellency, the Most Reverend Joseph T. McGucken, S.T.D.
Archbishop of San Francisco

Sister Mary Rose, Visitatrix, Daughters of Charity
Western Province

George L. Torassa, M.D., President, Mary's Help Hospital
Medical/Dental Staff

Sister Louise, Administrator, Mary's Help Hospital

DEDICATORY ADDRESS .... Honorable George B. Harris
Chairman, Mary's Help Hospital Lay Advisory Board

PLACING OF THE DEDICATORY PLAQUE AND
BLESSING OF THE BUILDING......................... His Excellency, The Most Reverend Archbishop Joseph T. McGucken, S.T.D.

EXPLANATION OF BLESSING .... Rev. Timothy E. O'Brien
Director of Health & Hospitals

Ave Maria—Soloist... Patricia Stolz

December 18. The dedication was held outdoors in what is now a parking area on the west side of the hospital. It is remembered as one of the coldest days on record. However, we had a very large, enthusiastic crowd caught up in the warmth of the ceremony and apparently unmindful of the weather.

Unfortunately it would be impossible to mention the names of all the people involved in the move. However, I would like to take this opportunity to acknowledge Sister Agatha Flynn. She was assigned to the old hospital in 1912 and served as Clinic Director and Pharmacist. On December 12, 1965, it was Sister Agatha who closed the door and turned the key on the old hospital when we moved. She and Jessie Miller, Director of Nursing Services, were the last two employees to leave the old hospital and join us at the new facility.

This seems to be the appropriate place to answer the question, "What was done with the old hospital building?" After we moved, the building was razed. A complex of 110 apartments for senior citizens, the Francis of Assisi Community, has been erected in its place. This

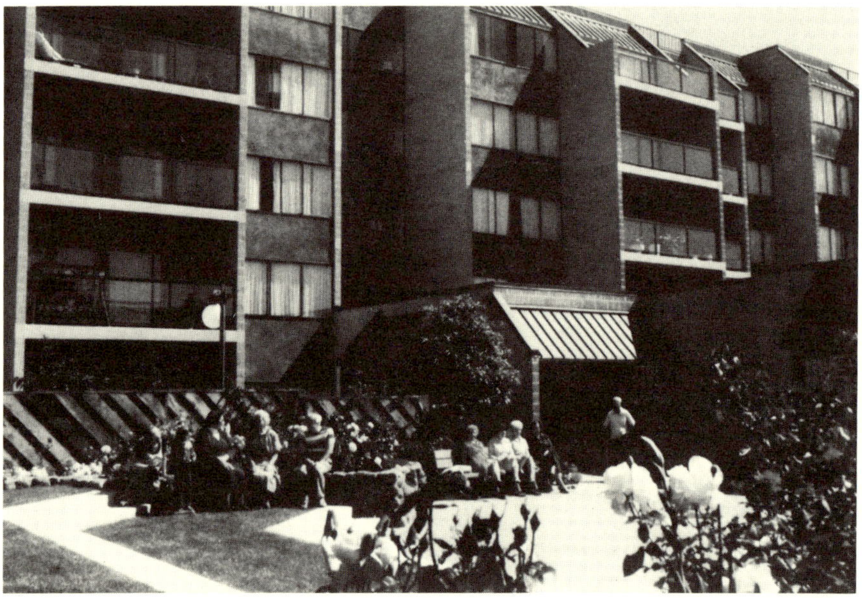

Francis of Assisi Retirement Residence, built on the site of the first Mary's Help Hospital at 145 Guerrero Street, San Francisco.

new building was dedicated on August 30, 1979 by Archbishop John R. Quinn and Archbishop Joseph T. McGucken. At present there are 115 residents there. Sisters Mariana Rabe and Lorraine Valdes served at Francis of Assisi Community for several years.

The following poem written by Josephine Knowles Smith, a resident of Francis of Assisi Community since its establishment in 1979, is testimony to the fact that the spirit and contributions of the Daughters of Charity remain at the Guerrero Street site.

I live in the Community of Francis of Assisi
where the first Mary's Help Hospital
used to be
sometimes I think I hear
the cry of a new-born babe
the nurses and doctors
moving from place to place
a bell for a priest
a Daughter of Charity
walking in the hall
whispering a prayer
yes—sometimes when I can't sleep
this is what I think I hear

there will always be
a Mary's Help Hospital
at 145 Guerrero Street
in the minds and hearts
of those who were born here
and those who owe their lives
to the care received here.

Preparing for the move was a happy and exciting time, but the memories are bittersweet. Mary's Help Hospital and its personnel suffered the loss of two of its most loved and respected people, Sister Andrea Neider and Tim McSweeney. The following special bulletin was issued by the employees of Mary's Help on November 5, 1965.

Sister Andrea, while she was not assigned to duty on a nursing station, was a prominent figure about Mary's Help. She arrived here in March 1962. From the day of her arrival, Sister's warm smile, keen sense of humor and her gentle and understanding ways made her a "house favorite." She was always seen traveling between the laundry or kitchen with an armful of clothing or food, for her responsibilities included the sewing for the Sisters and the management of their refectory.

Sister was quite a hand with a needle and thread; she worked long hours in preparing used clothing to be issued to her poor families. Her love for children is legendary; most of her Community life was spent either in orphanages or schools. No matter how busy she was, Sister Andrea could not resist stopping to chat with a child.

Sister Andrea loved a party! Who can forget how delighted she was to be present at the annual picnics to assist with the serving of the hot dogs at noon and seeing to it that everyone was amply fed at the evening meal.

Sister continued working up to the time she was last hospitalized on September 19th, and throughout her many long days of suffering she did not complain. She went to God quietly and happily on October 19, 1965. We know we have someone in Heaven praying for all of us!

Because of Sister Andrea's love for children, the personnel of Mary's Help have established a memorial fund in her name to provide some piece of equipment for Pediatrics. Contributions to the memorial may be made to Julia Golden (Admitting), Marie Abbruzzese (Library), or Jessie Miller (Nursing Service).

★ ★ ★

What can we say about Tim McSweeney? His forty-seven years at Mary's Help speak for his devotion and loyalty far more eloquently than words might.

Mr. Mc was a great-looking man with straight carriage, piercing blue eyes, and that gruff exterior. But underlying all of that was the heart of one of the kindest and most gentle men who ever lived. He could frighten you out of ten years' growth with one look—especially if he felt you had been responsible for causing any damage to "his Mary's Help." But if you looked deeply into his eyes you could see a devilish twinkle, and if you looked at his mouth, even in the midst of a tirade, you would have seen the corners curl in a smile.

Mr. Mc knew every pipe, every wire, every bolt and nail in Mary's Help. And God help you if you ever said an unkind word about the condition of the building.

Mr. Mc was a gentleman. He was an example of what every man could ever hope to be—a loving husband, a devoted father, a doting grandfather, a deeply religious man, a true friend. We'll miss that marvelous head of gray hair, the ever-present pipe, and that delightful brogue, but we know Mr. Mc is happy in having reached his final goal.

In Mr. McSweeney's honor, a memorial fund as part of the building fund has been established. Contributions may be made to this fund by contacting Joanne Curran (Clinic).

★ ★ ★

Their deaths at the height of our preparations bring to mind these lines from the *Rubaiyat* of Omar Khayyam.

Whether the Cup will sweet or bitter run,
The Wine of Life keeps oozing drop by drop,
The Leaves of Life keep falling one by one.

9

A New Beginning in Daly City 1966–1970

IN JANUARY 1966, the new hospital was flourishing. However, reaching the hospital was a problem. We were really isolated on the hill. The freeways were still only an engineer's dream. Nevertheless, services were established and employees adjusted very quickly to the new surroundings.

Although public transportation to the new hospital was not available at this time, car pools took care of the employees who did not drive. Actually, the number of employees lost to us because of the move was minimal. As of June 1985, 52 employees from Mary's Help in San Francisco were still with us at Seton Medical Center in Daly City.

As part of our plan to maintain the close "Mary's Help Hospital spirit" that was ours in the small hospital, Sister Justina Morgan, Councillor for Nursing, was requested to talk to all employees after we had arrived at the newer and larger facility. Sister had done this during the time of difficult decisions in San Francisco. Now she met in each department, all three shifts when necessary, to interact with all staff and convey in her unforgettable way the role of every employee. The staff had many requests for the prayer Sister Justina offered to open each session.

O Lord, My God, I undertake
this day's work alone in Your great name and for Your sake.
In ministering to suffering, I would learn
the sympathy and love that in Your Heart did burn.
For those who, on life's weary way,
unto disease diverse are prey,
Take, You, my eyes and teach them to perceive
the ablest way each one to receive.
Take, You, my hands, and in their touch may prove,
the gentleness and aptness born of love.

Take, You, my feet, and while they softly tread,
may I smile with understanding on every sufferer's bed.
Sanctify my lips and guide my tongue,
give me a word in season for each one.
All through the arduous day my actions guide.
Work through me, with me, in me, Lord, this day.

Mechanization at the new facility presented a challenge to us. The nurse-call system with audio at the nurses' station, the trayvayors, and the pneumatic tubes were a few of the new mechanized systems. We were accustomed to hand-delivery of supplies and equipment, and the change in Central Service—a completely automated system—required that we alter our ways.

The United States mail chutes on the nursing units were also new to us, and this was one change we all utilized enthusiastically. The difficulty was that they were not in official use for two months after they were installed, but we did not receive any notice from the Post Office. For a period, mail was deposited in the mail chutes on the nursing units and there it stayed. The Post Office did not pick it up. We realized what the problem was when we all began to receive notices about unpaid bills, inquiries from friends as to why we did not send Christmas cards, etc. The Post Office subsequently established the official use of these chutes.

This also brings to mind the transition from the old engine room at 145 Guerrero Street to the Engineering Department in Daly City. It was a tremendous change; we had entered the space age. Our long-term staff—Eddie Garcia, Hans Kraus and Tim Regan—met the challenge. In a short time they were able to operate or fix anything in the new facility just as they had been able to do at the old hospital.

The change from the old to the new laundry was a major one. But again our long-term Laundry Department employees mastered the complex machinery and new distribution systems without difficulty.

The weather in Daly City was another big change for us. We had come from the "sunshine-sheltered" Mission District of San Francisco to high on a hilltop in Daly City. The winter storms of January and February 1966 broke all records for this area. The winds gusts made entry and exit from the front and emergency entrances hazardous.

Personnel organized an escort service and continued this undertaking until adjustments in the entries were made. The wind also created problems with windows and the exterior light standards. The physical facility was really tested in our first months of occupancy. Emergency Department employees still relate stories about running out to the road to help patients and visitors enter and leave the building.

On November 21, 1966, we received an unexpected gift from the Macy Company. Sister Louise was notified she would be presented with the statue of the Madonna that is now in our lobby. The statue was carved of linden wood by Richard Lang of Oberammergau, a famous German master carver. A ceremony was quickly planned, and Sister made an impromptu acceptance speech.

The Emergency Department was busy from the day it opened, reflecting the need for an emergency service in the Daly City community. The Medical/Dental Staff rotated to provide coverage. This system continued for a few months. While the level of service and care was excellent, rotation was a hardship on the physicians. They were seeing patients with complaints very different from the patients they saw in their usual specialties. Thus, on March 28, 1966, an Emergency Department panel was created. The new system established physician coverage of the Emergency Department on a voluntary basis rather than the previous mandatory rotation system.

In April of 1966, we were selected by the magazine *Modern Hospital* for the Hospital of the Month Award. Certificates were presented to the hospital, the architects, the consultants, and the state Hill-Burton agency. *Modern Hospital*, August 1966, published the photos and the hospital design description.

By this time, the blue habit and white cornette worn by the Daughters of Charity for more than 300 years had been replaced by the present dark blue habit and simple coiffe. There is an interesting story that goes along with the origin of the first habit when the community was founded by St. Vincent de Paul in 1633 to care for the sick and the poor. The Daughters of Charity worked in homes as well as in hospitals. It was an idea whose time had come. There was a great need for an order of women to do this work, and young women from neighboring French villages responded in large numbers. Like women

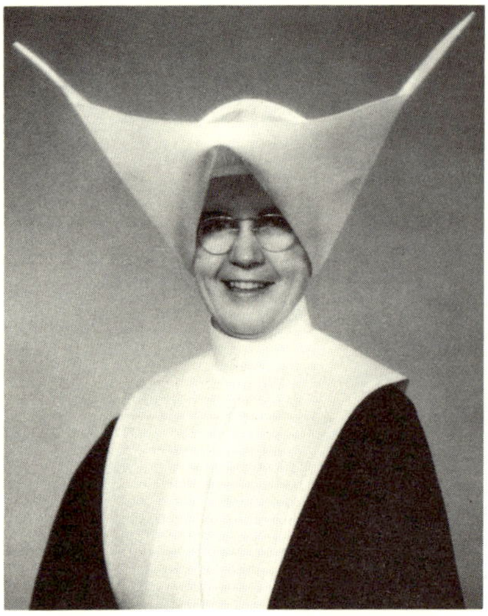

Sister Mary Rose McPhee
Habit prior to 1964

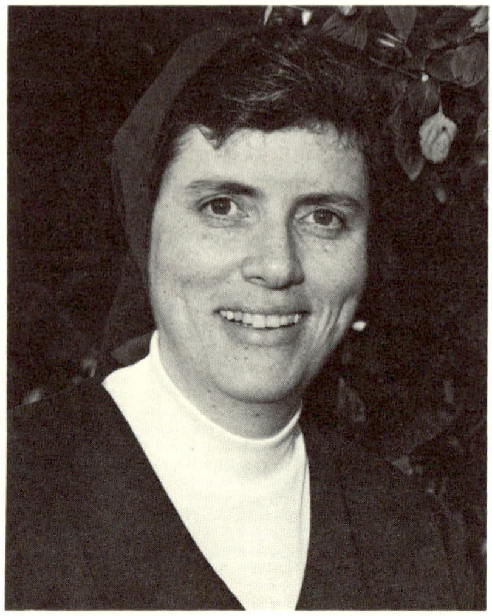

Sister Eileen Kenny
Current Habit

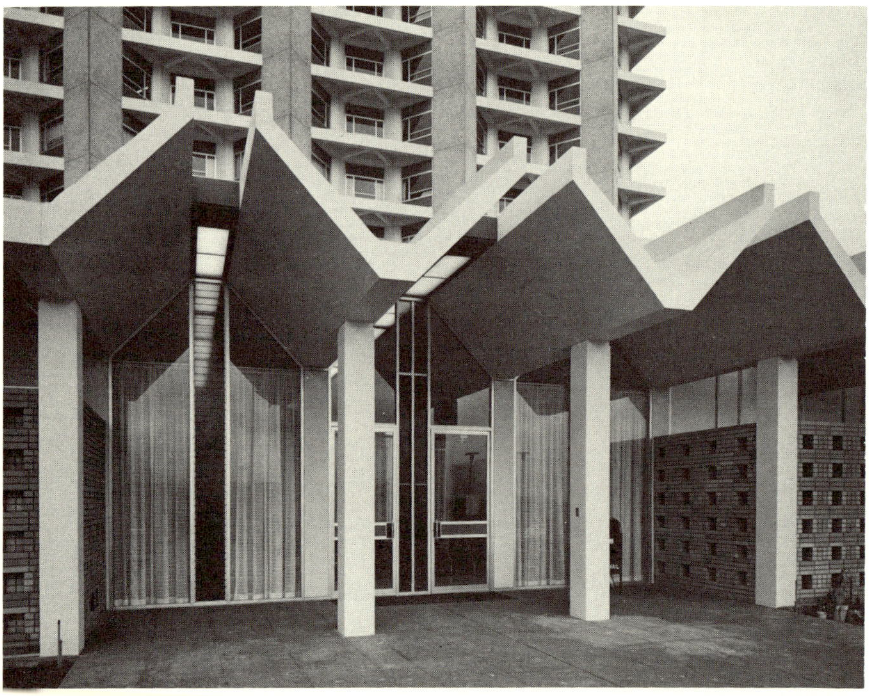

The facade of Seton Medical Center captures the design of the Daughters' cornette.

everywhere, their question to St. Vincent de Paul was, "What shall we wear?" St. Vincent, practical as always, said "Come as you are." So, the original habit was actually the French peasant dress of the seventeenth century. The facade of the present hospital's front entrance captures in stone the design of the Daughters' famous winged cornettes.

The design of the new hospital would probably be applauded by our first San Francisco benefactress, Mrs. Kate Johnson. A stipulation of her original endowment was that we build a "sunlight" hospital so that all patients might have the benefit of a view, the celestial dimension, and sunlight. Although the mandate did not have to be carried out in Daly City, it was. We are the "hospital with a view" in Daly City. The design of the building and the magnificent view from every window of the hospital are a tribute to the artistic talents of Sister Hermine Regan. The *Daughters of Charity Magazine*, Summer 1968, featured a pictorial series on the new hospital, which included the following description.

The Hospital with a View

Our views are multi-faceted—may we share them with you?
There is the "looking out" view from the windows of the hospital.
The views are shared by youth and age,
Their ills our challenge; their needs, our gauge.
There is the "looking in" view for all personnel of the hospital.
The view from within must be our age-old review.
The spirit of Charity each day born anew.
There is the "looking to" view for the residents of the surrounding area.
For those who look to us
The hospital is many things:
General services, emergency care,
The skillful hands that practice there,
A beacon of hope, staffed by those who care.
There is the "looking with" view for the Sisters and residents of surrounding communities.
As we join together to work and plan,
Our tasks encompass our fellow man;

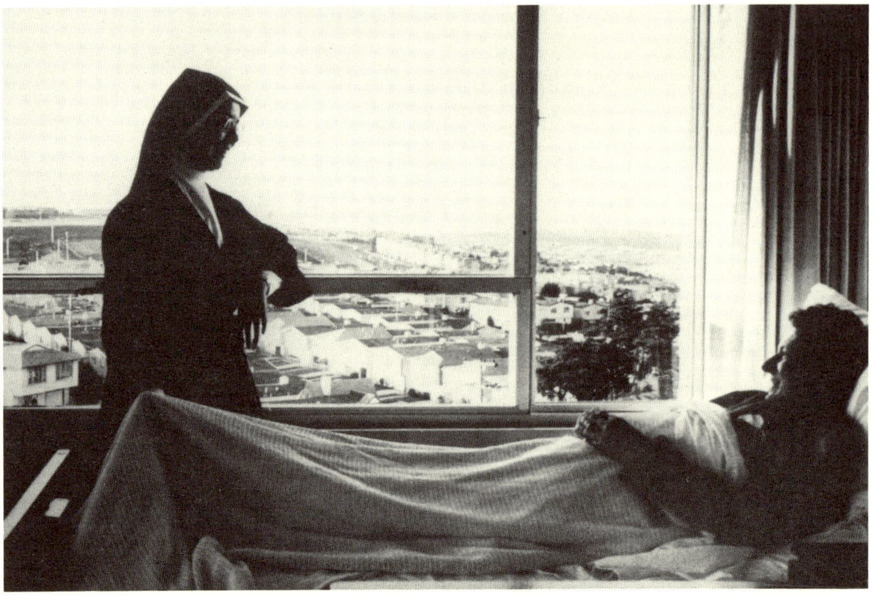

The "looking out" view from a patient's room in Daly City.

And in our efforts there emerges the view
Of a vision of charity—in all that we do.
There is the "looking ahead" view for hospital administration.
From history's pages the hospital is wrought;
Yet each day adjusts to new wisdom and thought.
The views are not limited by space or by time,
The dimensional depth and the vistas are wide.
For those who "look through" and those who "look to,"
Their view shall be hallowed by our love of mankind.

The hospital's occupancy rate and utilization of the Emergency Department increased steadily from 1966 to 1970. The upper three floors of the hospital were unfinished at this time, and consideration was given to completing them in order to provide more beds and services. Plans to utilize one unfinished unit, the eighth floor, began to emerge to satisfy the growing need for psychiatric services. The tenth floor was also a large open area, and was utilized at times as a wonderful roller-skating rink, notably by some Daughters of Charity!

In addition to growth in the clinical areas of the hospital, there were also significant developments in the non-clinical departments. Mary's Help was one of the first hospitals to form a hospital-wide education department. The philosophy of the Department of Education, which states our beliefs in relation to hospital education, follows:

> *We believe that man is a creature composed of body and soul substantially united and that he possesses gifts of intellect and free will, thus making him responsible to God for his acts. Mental, moral, spiritual, and physical rights are identical for every man regardless of race, creed, social and economic status.*
>
> *We believe that education is a dynamic process representing the sum total of the experiences, abilities, and potentialities of the individual throughout life.*

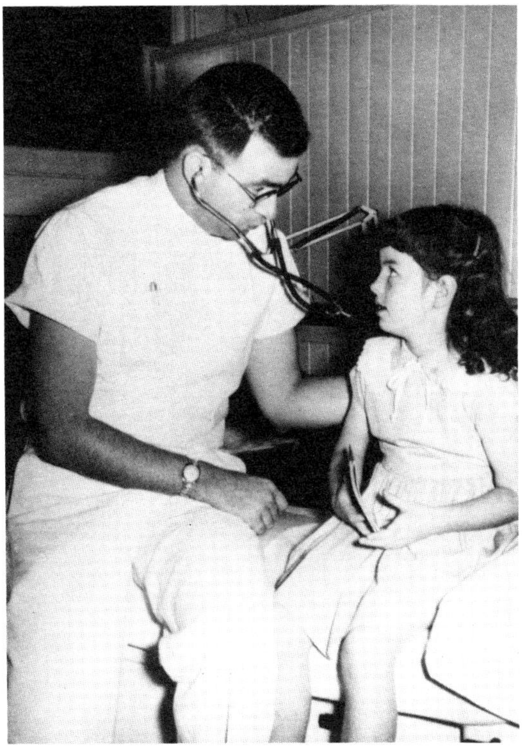

LeeRoy Eyheralde, R.N.
Offering patient education.

> *We believe that learning is a continuous process manifested by a change in behavior, and to become permanent it must be used in actual practice.*
>
> *We believe that hospital-based education is a part of adult education and requires structure and attention comparable to academic-based formal education.*
>
> *We believe that the opportunity to develop and improve competence of personnel at all levels and in all areas is an obligation of justice for hospitals because they render care through people.*
>
> *We believe education to be an integral part of the operation of a hospital because education is a change agent, and only people, personnel have the potential to appreciate—things depreciate.*

The role and significance of this department was well tested during the move and the settling-in process in the new hospital.

One of the Department of Education's earliest projects involved establishing a clinical experience program for various health professionals. Our first affiliating students were seniors from the School of Dentistry of the University of the Pacific in Stockton, California. This affiliation was an innovation in dental education because it provided students with a general hospital orientation and the opportunity to interact with the Medical/Dental Staff. This very successful affiliation was initiated by the Medical/Dental Staff President, George L. Torassa, Jr., M.D. and John P. Roffinela, D.D.S., Chief of the Division of Oral Surgery and Dentistry. Affiliating students from the nursing programs of the University of San Francisco, City College of San Francisco, and the University of California, San Francisco, and Radiology students from San Francisco City College also were at the hospital during this period.

As previously noted, our Clinic in San Francisco had closed on Tuesday, December 7, 1965. Without the benefit of an official opening, some of our Clinic patients made their way from San Francisco to the Emergency Department of the new hospital on the morning of December 13, 1965. They were treated there. In a short time our new Clinic services were established in the Emergency Department. The patient mix was both old and new, and the physicians giving their services were also old and new—some who served in the old Clinic in San Francisco and some who began in this new facility.

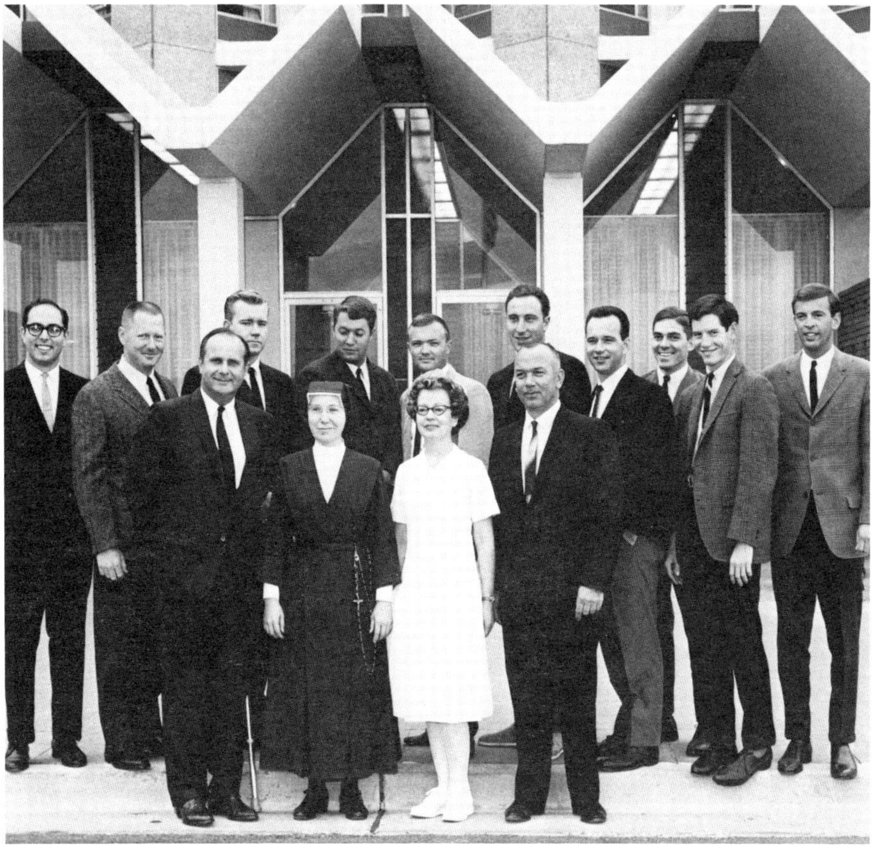

Dr. George Torassa, Jr., Sister Louise Scheessele, Marie Mahoney, and Dr. John Roffinela (front row), with affiliating students from the University of Pacific School of Dentistry.

Another very successful Department of Education activity was the parent education project, which came to be called "bench conferences." This series was developed for the Obstetrical Clinic patients. We found that these patients were not attending our weekly 7:00-9:00 p.m. parent education classes established in 1966 by Doctor Hubert Schwarz, Chairman of the Department of Obstetrics and Gynecology, and presented by the nursing staff of the Obstetrical Department. Upon investigation we learned that the reasons these patients did not come at night were lack of babysitters and lack of transportation. Our solution was to bring the classes to them as they waited in the Clinic area for their appointments with the obstetricians. The "bench conferences" were enthusiastically supported by the obstetricians, who adjusted their schedules to provide the patients medical appointments and classes in one visit to the hospital. Nursing students from the University of San Francisco made the "bench conferences" a class project. The students followed the patients when they were hospitalized and set up projects for obtaining layettes and other necessities.

During this time, the hospital's administration and the Medical/ Dental Staff planned yearly medico-legal moral seminars. Distinguished visiting faculties from medicine and law participated. Archbishop Joseph McGucken opened the first seminar in December 1966. Dr. George L. Torassa, Jr. was Program Chairman. The topics presented were:

THE PATIENT'S RIGHT TO KNOW
TRANSPLANTATION OF ORGANS
PERSONALITY DISORDERS
RESPECT FOR UNBORN LIFE
ORDINARY AND EXTRAORDINARY MEANS OF PRESERVING LIFE

Guest faculty members were Robert J. Barbieri, L.L.B.; Joseph J. Downing, M.D., Program Chief, San Mateo County Mental Health Service Division; J. Englebert Dunphy, M.D., Professor and Chairman, Department of Surgery, University of California School of Medicine; Donald C. Greaves, M.D., Professor and Head of Department of Psychiatry, University of Kansas School of Medicine; Emile F. Holman, M.D., Professor, Department of Surgery, Stanford University School of Medicine; Robert J. Luby, M.D., Associate Clinical Professor, Department of Obstetrics and Gynecology, Creighton University School of Medicine, Omaha, Nebraska; Rev. John J. Lynch, S.J., Professor of Moral Theology, Weston College, Weston, Massachusetts; and Leo O'Brien, L.L.M., School of Law, Gonzaga University, Spokane, Washington.

We celebrated our first birthday on December 12, 1966. Dr. George

L. Torassa, Jr., President of Medical/Dental Staff, wrote a note of thanks for the occasion:

To Those Who Have Served

The first 365 days have been an active, vigorous and exciting period. This past year has seen Mary's Help Hospital become an accepted and respected institution in its new location and a recognized and very important part of the medical community.

The success of this past year's operation has depended on many people and many departments. To mention a few: our housekeeping department has kept this hospital spanking-new and shiny as it was on the first day, and those in the laundry have made full use of their modern equipment in giving excellent service. There is hardly a patient who does not comment on the fine food and novel service of meals, all to the dietary department's credit. We should be aware that the engineering department has serviced and kept this huge plant running from the very first day without a major breakdown, which is remarkable for a first year's operation! The nursing department has worked night and day to give fine care to patients and service to doctors and has handsomely succeeded. This has been no small feat in view of events of the past year, and we are most grateful to our nurses and aides who showed themselves to be most faithful during the days of confusion.

Where do we begin and stop in this accolade? The girls at the switchboard are pleasant and efficient beyond compare. Our fine pharmacy and cooperative business office are most agreeable and helpful. The admitting and personnel departments and personnel must be thanked and congratulated. The medical records department is handling a herculean task with efficiency and under great stress, and yet is always courteous and ready to lend a hand.

In mentioning the nursing department, it goes without saying that all personnel in the clinic, emergency department and ICU are to be thanked and congratulated.

I know it is impossible to mention all who have given so much to making this first year successful but to each who reads this, technicians in pathology, surgery, x-ray, physiotherapy, and lay and professional members of this hospital in every area, all deserve to be praised and should have a feeling of satisfaction for the part they have played in the successful beginning history of Mary's Help Hospital in this new location.

One need only to mention the guild to be reminded of the tremendous good work and assistance it has given to the entire hospital.

The Medical/Dental Staff has been most active and has had continuing recognition throughout the year, reaching a peak with its seminar, "The Dignity of the Human Person." In March, the staff hosted and presented papers to the San Francisco Surgical Society.

Weekly rounds in the departments have had fine staff participation and attendance and during this year many outstanding speakers of national and worldwide reputation have come and made presentations at these meetings.

We all must give thanks to our chaplain, Father Francis Wajda, for his inspiration and continued spiritual guidance. We thank the Daughters of Charity and Sister Louise for making it possible for us to work together at Mary's Help.

In 1968, Mary's Help received from the Harney Foundation two separate donations of $100,000 in memory of the late Charles L. Harney. We owe these gifts to the generosity of the Foundation's President, Mrs. Charles L. Harney. One of the donations helped to build, furnish, and maintain the Clinic. The need for clinic services in the community and expansion of services was being studied at the time. The second donation was partially used for radioisotope laboratory equipment and an electromyograph. Charles L. Harney was a well-known San Francisco contractor, who was also a longtime friend of Mary's Help Hospital and served on the Advisory Board for many years. Not only did he make invaluable recommendations about maintaining the old facility, but he also guided us in hiring architects and selecting a site for the new hospital. We will remember him for his kindness and generosity, most of which was done very quietly.

Ours was the first Gastroenterology Laboratory in Northern

California. It was established in 1968 by Dr. Leo van der Reis, Chief of the Division of Gastroenterology. Since its origin, the services of the Laboratory have grown steadily. At the time of this writing, a full range of established gastrointestinal procedures, including laser technology, are performed in the Gastroenterology Laboratory.

During the construction, Sister Hermine mentioned to Dr. Charles Antonini, Sr., that she wanted to have a statue of the Sacred Heart of Jesus with outstretched arms placed in the main corridor of the hospital. The statue would be a symbol of hope and welcome to the patients, their families, and to all who would enter the hospital. Following this conversation, Dr. Antonini, while on a trip to Italy, ordered a statue of Carrara marble. The statue remains in the main corridor. It was the gift of Dr. Charles Antonini, Sr., in memory of his mother, Mrs. Catherine Antonini.

We also received the resignation of Judge George B. Harris, Chairman of the Community Advisory Board. The thirty-six member Community Advisory Board had been established in 1961 to plan the construction of the new hospital. Judge Harris chaired this committee for seven years. He guided the Board in the difficult times of fund raising and construction. In 1968, Judge Harris resigned from this position because of his increasing duties with the judiciary. In acknowledgment of his leadership and counsel, Judge Harris was unanimously awarded the office of Honorary Chairman of Mary's Help Advisory Board. Roy A. Bronson, senior partner in the law firm of Bronson, Bronson & McKinnon, and also charter member of the Advisory Board, was unanimously elected the new President.

A list of the Presidents of the Community Advisory Board follows.

George B. Harris	1961-1968
Roy A. Bronson	1968-1971
Carl E. Ward	1971-1973
Jack Hickey and Carl E. Ward, Co-presidents	1973-1976
Louis Cal LaLanne	1976-1979
Thomas Mellon	1979-1983
William E. McDonnell	1983-

The first focus of the Community Advisory Board was fundraising for the new hospital. Today, the Community Advisory Board is involved in additional projects. It remains concerned with construction problems and is also involved in finance and community needs that can be served by Seton Medical Center.

In August of 1968, we said good-bye to Sister Louise, who was assigned to Hotel Dieu of El Paso, Texas. It was Sister Louise, as Administrator, who provided the challenging leadership required for the move and the establishment of the new hospital. Sister Louise was replaced by Sister Teresa Piro who came to us from El Paso, Texas. Sister Teresa served as Hospital Administrator and subsequently was assigned a twelve-year term as Councillor for Health as a member of the first Provincial Council of the Province of the West. In February 1981, Sister Teresa was appointed Visitatrix (Provincial Superioress)

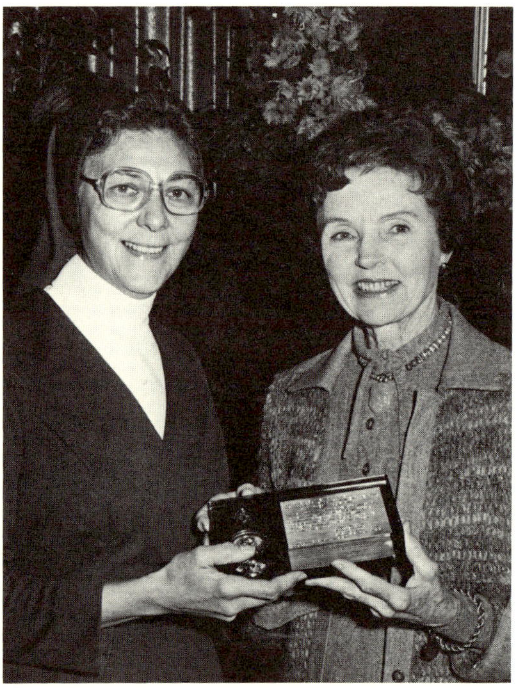

Sister Teresa Piro, Visitatrix of the Daughters of Charity, Province of the West, and Jane Wyatt.

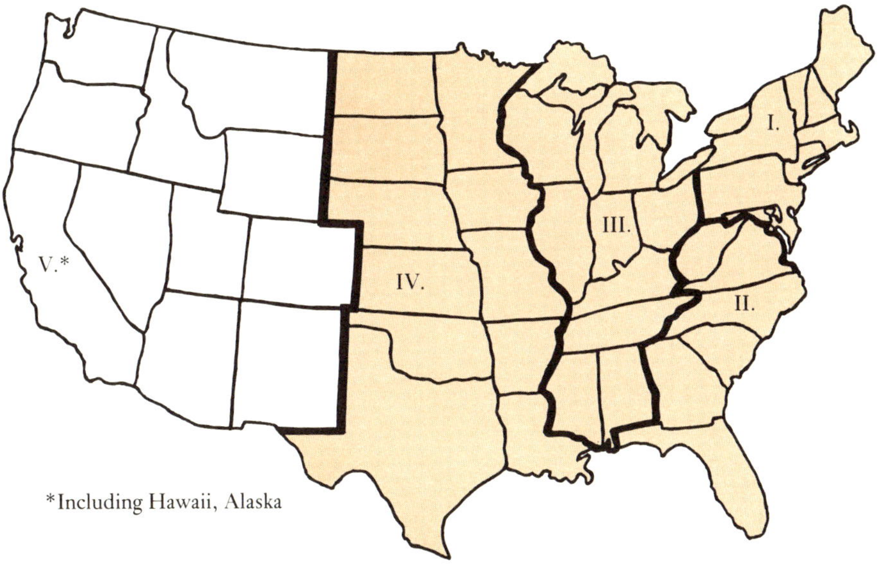

PROVINCES OF THE DAUGHTERS OF CHARITY OF ST. VINCENT DE PAUL IN THE UNITED STATES

I. North East Province
De Paul Provincial House
Albany, New York

II. South East Province
St. Joseph's Provincial House
Emmitsburg, Maryland

III. East Central Province
Mater Dei Provincial House
Evansville, Indiana

IV. West Central Province
Marillac Provincial House
St. Louis, Missouri

V. Province of the West
Seton Provincialate
Los Altos Hills, California

of the Daughters of Charity, Province of the West. She succeeded Sister Rose Collins, the first Visitatrix of the Province of the West. Sister Rose had served twelve years in this office; her vision, dedication, and assistance to Mary's Help Hospital was invaluable. Sister Teresa continues to provide support and motivation as the organization grows and adjusts to change in the health-care environment.

Until 1969 there were two provinces of the Daughters of Charity in the United States—one in the East and based in Emmitsburg, Maryland, and one in the West based in St. Louis, Missouri. The Daughters of Charity responded to growth by further division of the provinces. On January 4, 1969, the feast of St. Elizabeth Ann Seton, the two provinces were divided into five United States provinces. We became part of the Province of the West. At present the Province of the West has about 200 Daughters and 33 apostolic works in 6 states.

On March 31, 1969, Rex G. Chase was appointed Associate Administrator. Sister Teresa was Administrator at this time. There was a rapid succession of appointments for Mr. Chase. In March 1973 he became Administrator and in 1976, Executive Director. From January 1982 until his retirement in April 1985, Mr. Chase was President and Chief Executive Officer.

Frank C. Hudson, our current President and Chief Executive Officer, came to Mary's Help in September 1969 as Business Manager. He, too, had a rapid succession of promotions. He was Associate Administrator from July 1981 to August 1983, when he became Vice-president. In 1984 Mr. Hudson was appointed Administrator.

At the close of the 1960s Mary's Help Hospital was well established and recognized in Daly City and the surrounding communities. We were ready to enter into a period of rapid growth and expansion.

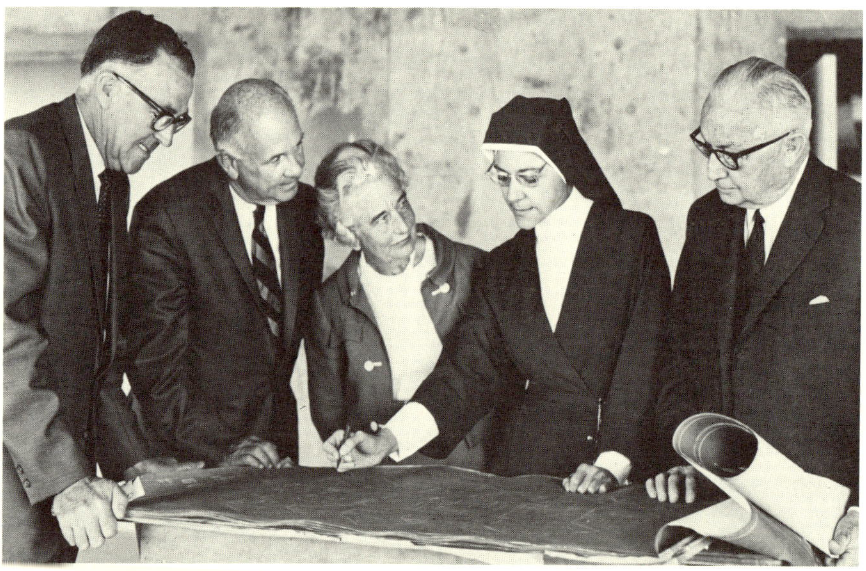

Planning for expansion: Jack Hickey, Henry Bostwick, Mrs. Ralph K. Davies, Sister Teresa Piro, and Roy Bronson.

10

Growth and Expansion 1970–1980

THE DECADE OF THE 1970S was one of great activity as Mary's Help Hospital responded to medical advances in the diagnosis and treatment of disease as well as to an increasing emphasis on wellness and prevention. Our significant growth in clinical areas was accompanied by advances in non-clinical areas and community outreach. It was the coalescence of a variety of activities that created the dramatic growth of this time.

At the suggestion of Sister Teresa Piro, who was then Councillor for Health, Province of the West, Sister Florence Urbine, who was at that time the Director of Education and Training at Saint Vincent Medical Center in Los Angeles, organized the Committee in Hospital-wide Education and Training for the Province of the West. She requested that Mary's Help Department of Education personnel participate. The purpose of this group was to share the ideas and projects of the Education Departments of Saint Vincent's Medical Center, O'Connor Hospital, and Mary's Help Hospital. Quarterly day-long meetings were held at each of the three hospitals on a rotating basis.

In 1970, the three hospitals sponsored workshops with the theme "Education—The Key to Untapped Potential." The objective of the sessions was to enable department managers from each hospital to meet and exchange ideas with their counterparts. This interaction reinforced the role and significance of hospital-wide education and also established open communication between the department managers of the hospitals in the Province of the West.

Many other activities of this period substantiate our commitment to education. We view education as an integral part of the entire hospital. It is something that transcends the organizational structure. In addition to the many hospital-wide and community education projects of this period, we were also committed to maintaining our medical education programs. The three-year Orthopedic residency training program was offered in conjunction with St. Joseph's and St. Mary's Hospitals. The combined rotating Orthopedic residency program was initiated by Dr. Merrill Mensor of Mary's Help Hospital, Dr. Lloyd Taylor of St. Mary's Hospital, and Dr. Ralph Soto Hall of St. Joseph's Hospital. We also had a one- or two-year surgical residency and a rotating intern program for General Medicine, Surgery, Pediatrics, and Obstetrics.

We were also affiliated with the University of the Pacific School of Dentistry and provided a course in Hospital Dentistry. This innovative program was designed to provide learning opportunities for the dentist in a general hospital. The dental student was also introduced to the clinical team concept—the role of the physician, dentist, and nurse in providing patient service and care.

SISTER ALICE MARY DEVINE
Providing pharmacy services for Clinic patients.

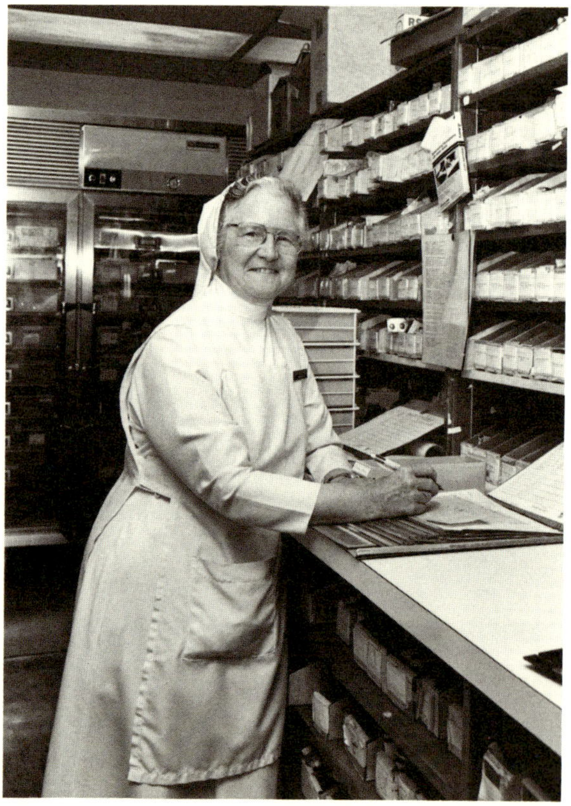

Ongoing clinical experience was provided for nursing students from baccalaureate programs at University of San Francisco, University of California, and San Francisco State University, as well as from the associate degree program of City College of San Francisco. We also offered clinical experience for radiology students from City College of San Francisco and respiratory therapy students from Skyline College of San Mateo.

When the hospital opened in 1965, the Outpatient Clinic, located on the first floor near the Emergency Department, offered clinic services to residents of both San Francisco and northern San Mateo Counties. Early in 1972, the Board of Directors approved a plan for further expansion and development of the clinic services. Implementation of the program began in August 1972. The hospital-based Clinic was relocated to the tenth floor, and outreach Clinics were established in Pacifica, San Bruno, and South San Francisco. Sister Arthur Gordon was in charge of the clinic services and directed the expansion program. During the following year the clinic medical services were expanded to include more than twenty-five specialties:

GYNECOLOGY

MEDICINE

- Allergy
- Cardiology
- Dermatology
- Gastroenterology
- General Medicine
- Internal Medicine
- Neurology
- Pulmonary Medicine

ORTHOPEDICS AND ORTHOPEDIC SURGERY

PEDIATRICS

- Free Immunizations
- Free Pre-School Examinations
- Free Well-Baby Clinic

SURGERY

- Cardiothoracic Surgery
- Ear, Nose and Throat
- General Surgery
- Neurosurgery
- Ophthalmology
- Oral Surgery and Dentistry
- Otology
- Plastic Surgery
- Proctology
- Urology
- Vascular Surgery

Each of the Clinics at Daly City, San Bruno, South San Francisco and Pacifica offered general family practice medical care to adults and children. Specialized care was provided at the hospital-based Clinic. The specialty Clinics were staffed by ninety members of the Medical/Dental Staff, who donated their services.

The hospital-based Clinic was in operation from 8:00 a.m. to 8:00 p.m., Monday through Friday. The bilingual outreach Clinics were also open in the evenings. Clinic visits increased from 2,100 patient visits for the fiscal year ending June 30, 1972 to almost 4,000 visits for the 1973 fiscal year.

The Clinics operated on a free or reduced-fee basis and were created to serve families or individuals who could not afford private medical care and who did not qualify for state-financed medical aid. Eligibility was determined on a sliding scale of income depending upon the number of family members.

Mary's Help Hospital expanded its charity service in 1972, when we first provided medical care through the Flying Samaritans clinics. Flying Samaritans is a non-profit, private charitable organization that provides medical assistance to individuals living in remote areas. Volunteer doctors, nurses, and other professionals visit Flying Samaritans clinics in Northern California (where there are many American Indians living in the Trinity Alps) and in the Mexican states of Sinaloa, Sonora, and Baja California. The Flying Samaritans also travel to other locations for consultations, emergencies, and special clinics. When it is required, they bring patients to hospitals in urban areas.

Dr. Paul Pitlyk and a number of physicians, nurses, and other Mary's Help Hospital professionals participated in this service. They flew to remote areas and established local clinics or transported the patients to the hospital when surgery or other special services were required.

In the summer of 1973, the unfinished eighth floor was completed. A thirteen-bed Mental Health Unit, which offered inpatient psychiatric services and twenty-four-hour emergency mental health care, admitted its first patients. The facility was designed to be a short-term treatment center. It was partially funded by a grant, awarded in 1972

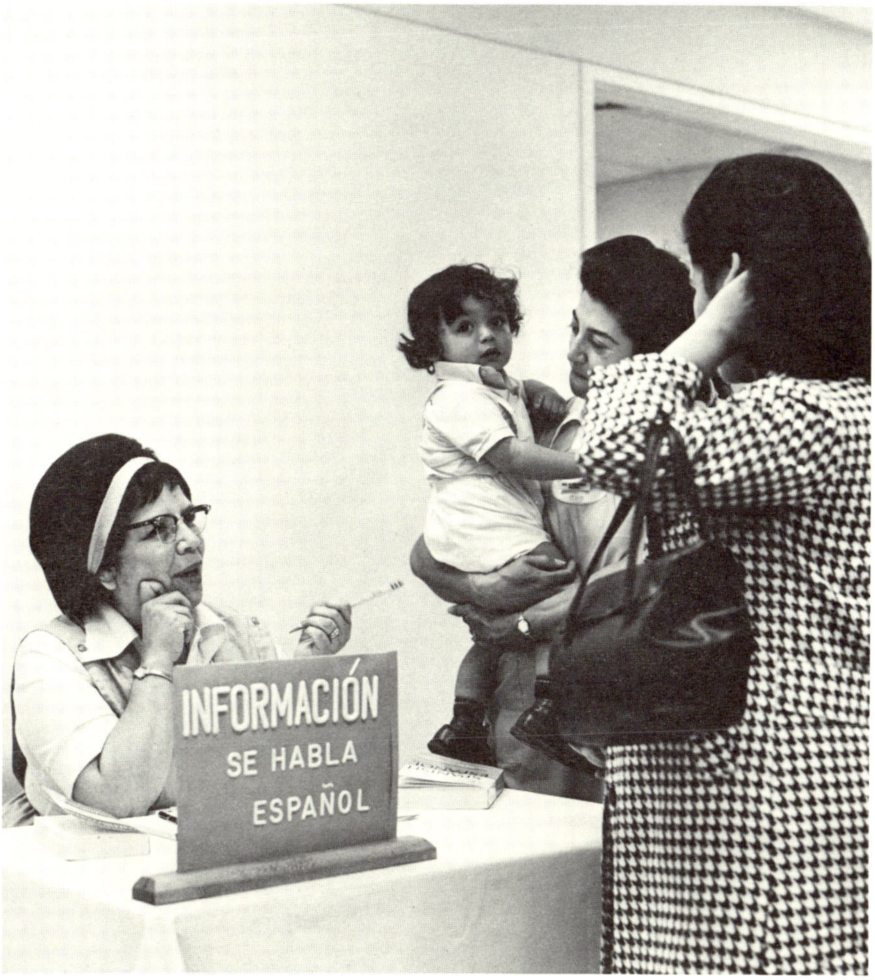

At one of Mary's Help Hospital's bilingual outreach clinics.

by the National Institute for Mental Health (NIMH). Margaret K. Sainio, M.D., PhD., was the first Director of the Division of Psychiatric Medicine. In January 1984, George Bach-y-Rita, M.D. became Director.

In September 1973, six beds were added to the Mental Health Unit, bringing the total to nineteen. In October 1975, outpatient psychiatric services were initiated to provide counseling and mental health care to

Clinic members and former hospital patients. Psychiatric social workers provided this service at the hospital and outreach Clinics.

In May 1973, Sister Florence Urbine was appointed to the Board of Directors, and in 1974 became President of the Board. Shortly after her appointment as President, Sister Florence announced plans for expansion of the hospital's support departments.

Statistics reinforced the need to expand the ancillary services. In 1968, there were 16,000 patients treated in the Emergency Department; in 1973, there were 27,000. Since 1969, Laboratory visits were up 51 percent, Radiology visits increased 49 percent, and Physical Therapy visits were up 47 percent. The number of surgeries increased 29 percent.

Financial assistance for the construction came from several sources. A voluntary capital fund drive was launched by civic leaders who formed an Expansion Fund Executive Committee. They were Gerson Bakar, Henry Bostwick, Mrs. Ralph K. Davies, Brig. General Arthur

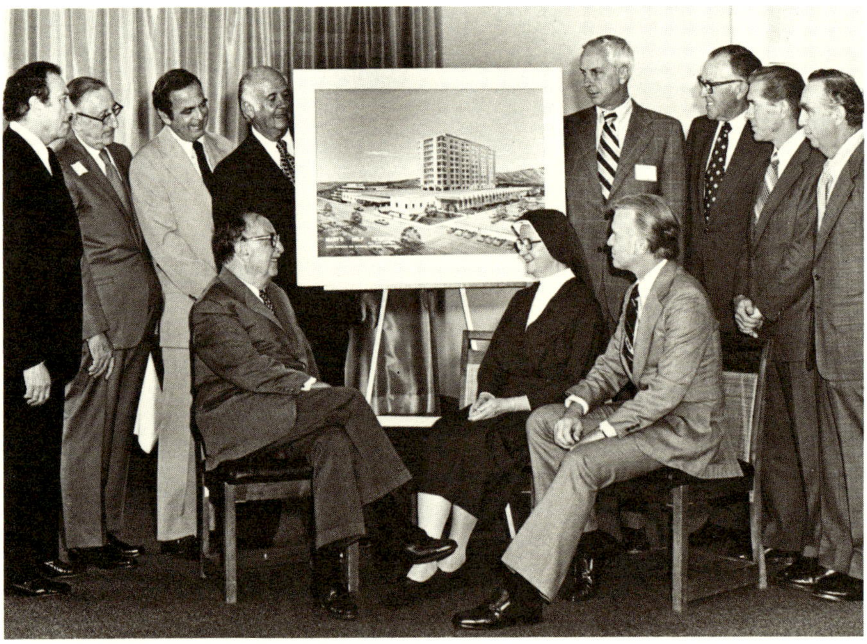

Sister Florence Urbine, Chairman of the Board of Directors, with the Expansion Fund Executive Committee.

H. Frye, Jr., Jack Hickey, Thomas J. Hunter, Robert L. Follet, Edward M. King, Edmund T. King, General Andrew Lolli, F. D. Minucciani, Frank Pacelli, W. C. Scollin, Charles Turner, Carl Ward and Benjamin H. Swig, Chairman. The Medical/Dental Staff campaign was co-chaired by Drs. William Dowling and Beth Reimer. The Mary's Help Hospital Guild pledged $300,000, and the employees raised $82,000 themselves in a week-long campaign.

We also began construction on two other separately financed projects that were not part of the expansion program. They were the Sisters' home and the professional office building.

On May 29, 1974, Dr. Robert A. Bilafer, President-elect of the Medical/Dental Staff, died suddenly. During his forty-year association with the hospital, he had been elected both in 1957 and in 1974 as President of the Medical/Dental Staff. He served on virtually every medical staff committee. In 1957, he was selected by Archbishop John J. Mitty to replace Dr. Alexander S. Keenan on the Board of the Corporation. Dr. Bilafer served on the Board until 1963 when the control of the Corporation was transferred to the Community of the Daughters of Charity.

In June 1974, the registered nurses, as members of the California Nurses Association, struck against the Affiliated Hospitals of San Francisco. (We are still considered a San Francisco hospital because of our membership in the Affiliated Hospitals.) The strike continued for over three weeks. During this period, all hospital services remained open. Nursing care was provided by nurses who usually worked in administrative positions and by nursing assistants, who provided tremendously helpful support. We had additional help from the Daughters of Charity. With the nursing hours rearranged to the old twelve-hour shifts—day nurses 7:00 a.m. to 7:00 p.m., night nurses 7:00 p.m. to 7:00 a.m.—we managed to maintain our standard of care. Thanks to the cooperation of all on the ninth floor and the third floor, managed by nurses from the Department of Education, we were able to establish daily in-service education on the units during this period!

I learned a very valuable lesson about priorities during the strike. My assignment was medicine nurse on the ninth floor and later on the third floor. Early one morning I received a message from Mr. Chase, the Administrator, requesting that I attend a very important 10:00 a.m. meeting for department managers. Without the slightest hesitancy I answered, "Tell Mr. Chase I'm giving medicines and can't come." This was out of character for me, as I normally responded to the Administrator, and in the Department of Education we were always calling people to attend meetings and classes. But during the strike my top priority was administering medications correctly and on time. I would let nothing else interfere. Actually, I thought no more about it. That night at about 6:15—by then I was on the 6:00 p.m. medicines— Mr. Chase and Sister Frances McCarthy, a member of the Provincial Council and Assistant to the Visitatrix, came to the unit with the greeting, "Well, as you wouldn't come to us, we thought we would come to you." That night I achieved greater tolerance and understanding of the priorities of others.

In April 1975, we participated in "Operation Baby Lift," a program sponsored by the State Department to airlift orphans out of war-torn Vietnam. An area of the Pediatrics unit was specially prepared for the orphans. The Sisters and employees provided clothes and toys for the infants. The children, who ranged in age from two months to two years old, were treated for skin infections, vitamin deficiencies, pneumonia, diarrhea, chicken pox, and other children's diseases. Following treatment they were sent to their new homes. Mary's Help Hospital cared for more Vietnamese orphans during "Operation Baby Lift" than any other hospital in the Bay Area.

September 1975 was a month of celebration for the Daughters of Charity and Mary's Help Hospital. On September 9, 1975, Mother Seton was canonized in Rome. More than 100,000 people, including 20 Daughters of Charity from the Province of the West, attended the ceremony presided over by Pope Paul VI in St. Peter's Square in Rome. On September 20, 1975, Archbishop Joseph McGucken presided at a Mass at St. Mary's Cathedral in San Francisco. Throughout the month there were receptions for all employees. Highlighting the program was a display depicting events in the life of Elizabeth Bayley

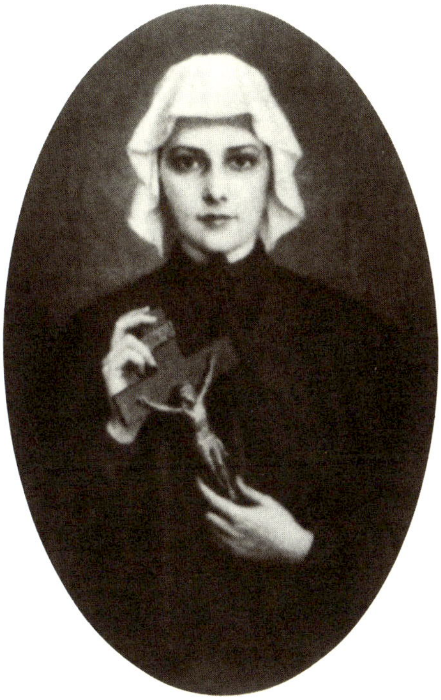

ST. ELIZABETH ANN SETON
First American woman to be canonized (September 1975).

Seton. She was the first native-born American woman to be canonized in the Roman Catholic Church and became Saint Elizabeth Ann Seton, the American foundress of the Daughters of Charity.

In June 1975, Sister William Eileen Dunn was appointed our first Patient Advocate. She was followed by Sister Mary Helen Doerr, who continued to develop the role and responsibilities of this new position. The Patient Advocate assists patients with non-medical problems and provides general information about the hospital and related services. From the first Patient Advocate to the present one, Sister Kathleen O'Sullivan, a comprehensive analysis of each patient's perception of and responses to our care has been developed. The patient questionnaire in current use is recognized as a valuable source of information about the effectiveness of the hospital services.

A natural family planning center was opened in late October 1975 with an introductory class in the Billings ovulation method of family planning. The course is now offered for three weeks—or six sessions. Classes are open to the public. The ovulation method of family planning was developed by the husband-wife team of Australian physicians, John J. and Evelyn Billings. The Billings method is a simple, accurate method of birth regulation that does not involve any drugs or the use of any instrumentation. The method can be used both to achieve or to avoid pregnancy. It is taught in the natural family

SISTER
WILLIAM EILEEN DUNN
Our first patient advocate

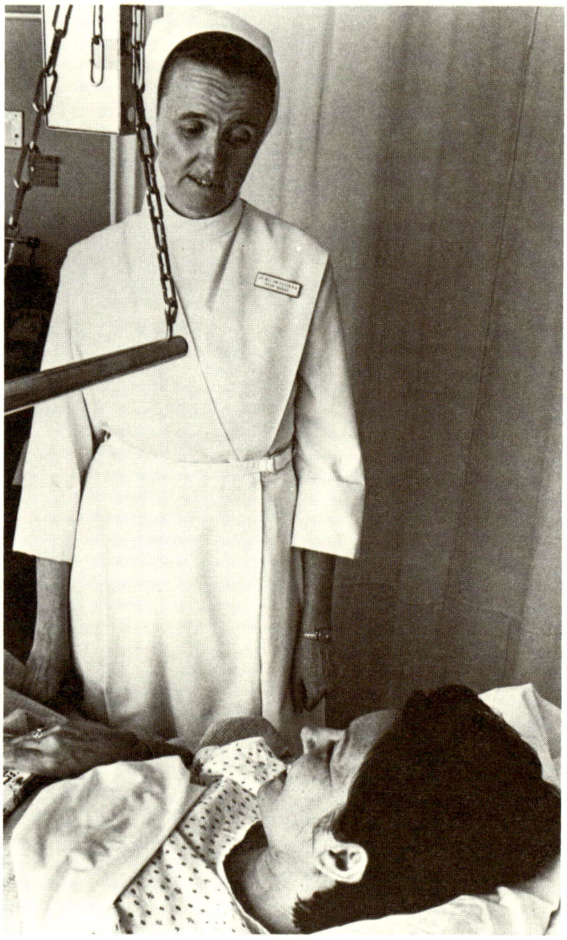

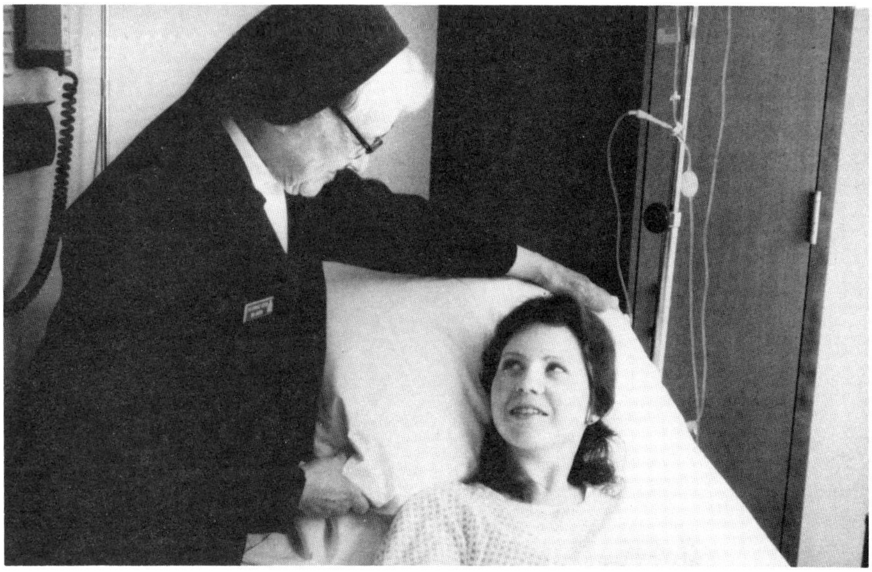

Sister Carmen Ptacnik of Pastoral Care keeps the department's tradition that each patient will be visited each day by a Sister.

planning centers that have been established in several major metropolitan areas throughout the United States. Molly Woerner, who remains an instructor, established our program, which is sponsored by the Archdiocese of San Francisco.

Two departments of the hospital particularly expressive of the mission of the Daughters of Charity—Social Service and Pastoral Care—were very active in this period. Social Service was organized as a department in 1923 in San Francisco, and the role and range of services has expanded in Daly City. The Department of Pastoral Care was established to highlight the recognition given to pastoral care as an integral department within the wholistic approach to health. The Daughters of Charity assigned to the Pastoral Care Department have been able to maintain our tradition that each patient will be visited by a Sister each day. Sister Sharon McCarthy is the present Director.

Tele-Care was established in this decade by the Guild and is now one of its most active programs. Daily phone calls are made to the elderly who live alone or are incapacitated. If the phone call is not answered, a back-up person is notified, and the calling continues until contact is made. The service has been a life-saving one for people who have had medical emergencies while they were alone. The Tele-Care volunteers make the calls every morning, including weekends and holidays. The service is available in foreign languages as well as in English. There is no charge for the service, and the public is invited to participate.

Work on the modernization and expansion project of the hospital began in 1976. An environmental impact report and a zoning plan were approved by the City Council of Daly City and a building permit was issued. The California Department of Health authorized the start of construction.

The expansion projects included the building of three critical care units. The new Carl Gellert Ambulatory Care Center was built in response to the trend in the health-care industry away from hospitalization and toward ambulatory care, which substantially lowers the

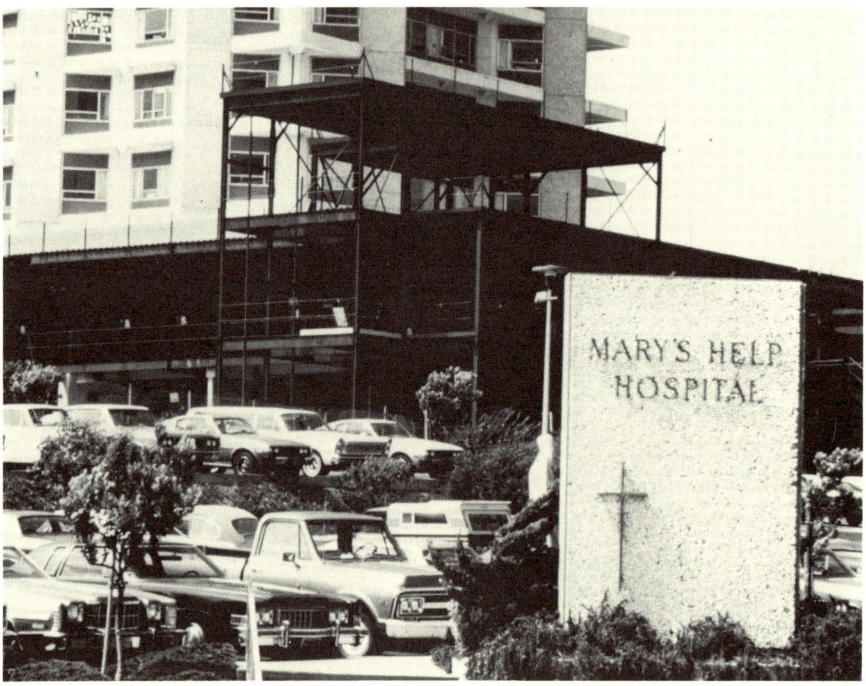

Work on the modernization and expansion project began in 1976

cost of patient care. A physiological testing center was also created to centralize several services and departments, such as EEG, EKG, EMG, gastroenterology, pulmonary function testing, and outpatient respiratory therapy.

The modernization and expansion project also included plans for Cardiovascular Surgery facilities, a Cardiac Catheterization Laboratory, a Radiation Therapy Department, and a computerized axial tomography (CAT) scanner.

When the project was completed, Mary's Help Hospital had a "new look." The original building—the tower—is now surrounded by two- and three-storied additions, or pods. A unique feature of the expansion is the extension of the hospital building to the east, which provides access to the building at a sub-ground floor level. Due to the natural slope of the terrain adjacent to the new entrance, there are elevators connecting the lower level with the ground and first floors.

Each year the Emergency Department sees an increasing number of patients with a growing range of medical problems. In 1976, San Mateo County contracted with Medevac for a fleet of paramedic-staffed ambulances to service emergency calls throughout the County.

In 1977, Mary's Help, Mills and Sequoia Hospitals were selected by the San Mateo County Board of Supervisors as emergency service base stations. The physicians who have staffed the Emergency Department since February 9, 1978 are all specialists in Emergency practice and are members of the California Emergency Physicians. Members of our Medical/Dental Staff serve on referral panels for additional consultation in the care of emergency patients.

The specially trained paramedics become the eyes and ears of the physician when they are at emergency sites. Physicians and nurses at the technically equipped Emergency Department can direct the paramedics at an accident site, via radio, in the administration of advanced life support functions. The radio network between physician and nurse emergency specialists provides both voice and biomedical telemetric communication. The radio link allows physicians and nurses in designated Emergency Departments to serve as base stations for paramedic supervision and to direct emergency medical care with

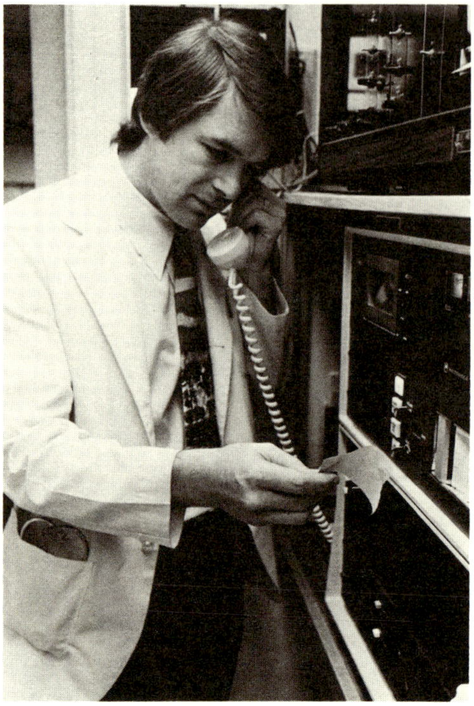

An Emergency Department physician talks by radio with a paramedic at the scene of an accident.

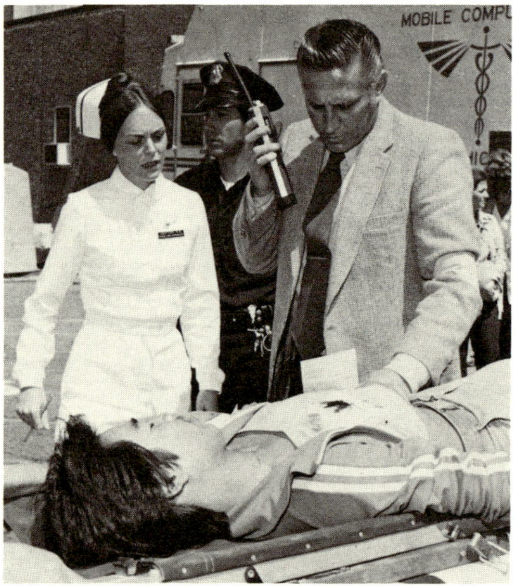

Judy Cook, R.N., and Donald Wald, M.D., participate in an emergency disaster drill.

knowledge of the patients' condition. For example, the transmission of an EKG reading might indicate to a physician at the Emergency Department that a patient at the site of an accident is experiencing cardiac arrhythmias and that immediate defibrillation by the paramedic is indicated to sustain life.

Since we are an emergency base station, all ambulance patients in northern San Mateo County are monitored by our personnel until they arrive at a hospital. When we are not the receiving hospital, our Emergency physicians and nurses will telephone ahead to the receiving hospital. All ambulance runs are documented and serve as evidence of medical supervision and paramedic intervention. The information is also used in future education sessions.

Continuing education of paramedics, registered nurses, and other Emergency personnel is one of our major responsibilities as a base station. Professional nurses in the Emergency Department are required to be certified as mobile intensive care nurses. They must enroll in a theory course and accompany paramedics on six simulated runs and six actual emergency runs. They must also pass the San Mateo certification examination.

Although it was in the latter part of the seventies that we began special cardiac procedures and cardiac surgery, our involvement in the medical treatment of heart disease has a long and significant history. Dr. Albert C. Reed was one of the founders of the Cardiac Clinic program in the Depression era. He was later joined by Dr. Francis Rochex. The Cardiac Clinic was a very active service, and their work attracted Bay Area cardiologists to their monthly luncheon meetings. These educational sessions, chaired by Dr. Rochex, had an average attendance of fifty cardiologists and continued until the physicians left for military service in World War II.

We spent several years preparing for the development of present cardiac services at Mary's Help. The plans involved cooperation of many experienced professionals in a series of seminars, clinical training sessions, and travel to other hospitals. Upon completion of personnel training, specially trained nurses, anesthesiologists and perfusionist technologists joined the cardiovascular surgeons of the Mary's Help Hospital Medical/Dental Staff to make up our heart team.

Mary's Help then established fully equipped Cardiac Care and Transitional Care Units with telemetric monitoring equipment for post-cardiac surgical patients.

The Cardiac Catheterization and Special Procedures Laboratory opened in December 1977. The hospital's first coronary artery bypass operation was performed by Dr. Merrill Bronstein on February 13, 1978. Dr. Elias Hanna also began coronary bypass and heart valve replacement surgery here. These events marked our entrance into the operative treatment of heart disease.

The success of any cardiovascular surgery program is dependent upon the support of a number of hospital services, notably the Departments of Radiology, Anesthesiology, Nuclear Medicine, Respiratory Therapy and the Laboratory.

On May 1, 1978, we had a strike. Physicians in Northern California hospitals scheduled a work stoppage to protest the tremendous increase in their malpractice insurance rates. Our plan of action during this period differed from that of several San Francisco hospitals. For example, in San Francisco an emergency anesthesiologist could provide anesthesia and transport the patient after surgery to the county hospital for follow-up care. At Mary's Help, our anesthesiologists also rendered services only in cases of emergency, but the patients were not transferred to other hospitals. We maintained compliance with our approved policies on the transfer of patients.

Most hospital services operated normally (although at a reduced level) throughout the malpractice insurance crisis. The main exception was reduced anesthesia for elective surgery. However, patient occupancy rates dropped 25 percent at the height of the crisis, causing the hospital to lose an average of $12,000 per day in patient revenues. This was partially offset by reductions in personnel costs and other expenses. In response to the decreased census, 92 Mary's Help employees were temporarily laid off due to the effects of the malpractice crisis. Many employees simply took early vacations or leaves of absence without pay during the work stoppage, resulting in an overall 18.5 percent reduction in staff.

In the summer of 1978, there were a number of additions to our maternity services. Anne Garrett, R.N. and Mary Steinhauer, R.N. started a new childbirth health education series for the community. The classes prepare couples for childbirth by providing the information they need to actively participate in the experience of pregnancy and childbirth. Couples may enroll in one or more of the courses and are not required to schedule delivery at the hospital. While the majority of participants do deliver here, some choose to deliver at other hospitals in San Francisco or San Mateo. The classes are, however, a prerequisite for giving birth in our Alternative Birth Center (ABC).

Natural childbirth in the hospital setting became a reality in September 1978, with the opening of the Alternative Birth Center. Dr. Norman Wheeler, Chairman of the Department of Obstetrics and Gynecology, introduced the new service:

> *Parents have the chance to make childbirth an event both family and close friends can share, just as they did before hospital births*

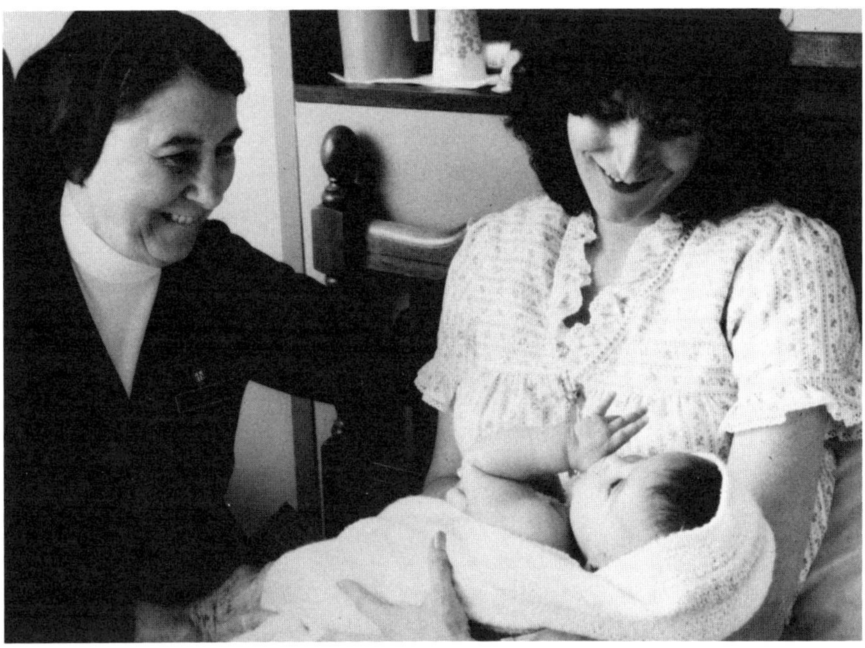

Sister Paula Landry visits employee Sandra Pieschel and her new daughter Amanda.

became the general rule. Unlike mothers of a century ago, mothers today need not risk dangers from natural childbirth because all the resources of modern medicine are only steps away from the ABC in the event of an emergency.

Natural birth, he stressed, is for the low-risk mother, and the determination is made by her personal obstetrician. Susan and Larry Thompson were the first couple to have their child in the Alternative Birth Center. Stacey, their six-pound, five-ounce baby daughter, was born on September 29, 1978.

In 1979, the inventors of the CAT scanner (computerized axial tomography) were awarded the Nobel Prize for Medicine. Later that same year we completed our plans to acquire a scanner. The origin of this tremendous technology goes back to November 1895 and to the work of Wilhelm Conrad Roentgen, Professor of Physics at the

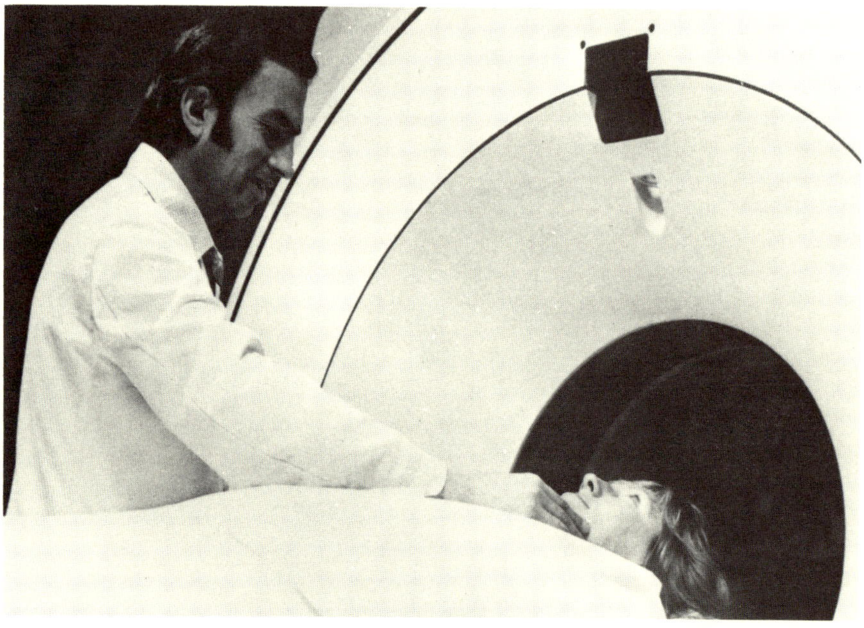

Oscar Guzman, CT Technologist, operating the CAT scanner acquired in 1979 by the Radiology Department.

University of Würzburg, Germany. With the invention of X-rays it was possible for the first time to visualize the bones and the body cavities. Shortly after the introduction of X-rays came the discovery of radioactivity of uranium by Becquerel and isolation of the element radium by Pierre and Marie Curie. Thus, the "new" science of radiology was born almost a century ago.

Pioneers in Radiology would be astonished at the quantum leap in diagnostic capability made possible by the combination of computers and X-rays in computerized tomography. This modality permits physicians to visualize internal portions of the body that have not been possible to view with conventional X-rays. The CAT scanner also detects much more subtle differences in tissue density than had been previously possible. The radiologists now have a new major diagnostic tool at their command.

A significant development in Radiology at Mary's Help Hospital was due to the work of Dr. Alexander Petrilli, Director of the Department of Radiology. He was an early leader in creating the techniques used in mammography. Dr. Petrilli served at the hospital for twenty-five years.

The fifty-five-million dollar construction program and the multifaceted growth of Mary's Help Hospital progressed rapidly during the close of this decade.

II

The Present 1980–1985

OUR HISTORY has been shaped by a pattern of growth and change. The years 1980 to 1985 are characterized by a rapidly changing health-care environment. We find ourselves facing financial and regulatory constraints. While these constraints have presented problems, they have also stimulated new and innovative approaches to the delivery of health care.

As I reflect upon the kaleidoscope of events that make up our history, I realize that the mission of our sponsor, the Daughters of Charity of St. Vincent de Paul, is the linchpin of all our activities. The mission is constantly reinforced in attitude and in practice. It is our ongoing commitment to integrate our strategic business plans with our spirit and philosophy that unites us.

The Board of Directors of the hospital was determined that the values set forth in the Daughter's mission be recognized and in place as we faced the changes the eighties would bring. In 1979, the Board requested the formation of a hospital-wide Organizational Steering Committee. The charge given the Committee was to identify those programs and activities that were designed to communicate the culture and influence the organizational climate. The Board also specified that the degree of employee involvement in these activities be included in the report.

In January 1980, Frank C. Hudson, Administrative Coordinator for Organization Development, presented the Organization Steering Committee's Plan of Action to the Board of Directors. The Committee recommended that a program be created to manifest more clearly our mission and purpose as a Catholic health-care facility. The Board of Directors accepted the Plan of Action with the recommendation that the Committee direct itself toward the changes in cultural and organizational values set forth in the plan. There were several specific shifts in cultural and organizational values that the Board supported. The following schema illustrates the changes sought.

VALUE SHIFTS RECOMMENDED IN THE PLAN OF ACTION

CULTURAL VALUES

FROM		TOWARD
Independence	→	Interdependence
Endurance of Stress	→	Capacity for Fulfillment

ORGANIZATIONAL VALUES

FROM		TOWARD
Technological Mode	→	Humanistic Mode
Competitive Relations	→	Collaborative Relations
Separate Objectives	→	Linked Objectives
Department Resources Regarded As Owned Absolutely	→	Department Resources Regarded As Organization's Resources
Acceptance of Work as a Means of Survival	→	Awareness of Work as a Participation in God's Activity
Intellectual Recognition of Acceptance of Gospel Values	→	Implementation of Gospel Values in Operation of the Total Organization, Each Department, Each Position

The Board of Directors then set up a series of workshops in which they reviewed the Philosophy Statement of the Health Apostolate of the Province of the West and drafted the Mission and Goal Statements of the hospital. Following the workshops, the Board members presented these documents to the administrators and department managers in a number of education sessions. It then became our charge to develop a program that would communicate the message of these documents to all involved in any way with the organization. It was Sister Marilynn Emminger, now Health Councillor, Province of the West, who provided the motivation and support as we worked to create a plan and process to communicate our identity and values.

The program we developed is called *Vincentian Values*. The first class was held in April 1981. It is still offered today in all departments, on all shifts, and to community groups. To date, more than 3,000 people have participated. We have achieved an extensive outreach for the *Vincentian Values Program*. It received honorable mention from the Catholic Health Association Achievement Citation Program in 1984 and 1985. Due to this publicity many Catholic health facilities throughout the United States request the use of the program, which was copyrighted in 1984.

An abbreviated outline of the current five-phase program follows.

Plan of the Vincentian Values Program

PHASE I EDUCATION	This phase provides the cognitive base of the philosophy, mission and goals of Seton Medical Center.
PHASE II ASSIMILATION	This phase provides opportunities for validation and implementation of each department's philosophy in conjunction with the study of the philosophy of Seton Medical Center.
PHASE III INTEGRATION	This phase creates a plan of action for departmental implementation of the goals of Seton Medical Center. The plan is updated yearly.
PHASE IV EVALUATION	This phase utilizes the Catholic Evaluative Criteria Program to evaluate the Vincentian Values Program as it is implemented at the operations level. This evaluative process provides a foundation for the integration of Gospel values and the healing ministry of Jesus into the entire organization on a corporate level and into the performance expectations of each employee.
PHASE V RENEWAL	In this phase, the Board of Directors will examine and update the Mission and Goal Statements. The Board will consider the impact of the program on the organization. They will also evaluate the shift from intellectual recognition of Vincentian Values to their implementation in operation throughout the organization.

The integration model from the program was incorporated in the Strategic Business Plan of Mission Services Corporation in 1983. This event supports the degree to which the *Vincentian Values Program* has infiltrated the hospital and our subsidiaries.

Model Showing Need for Integration of Strategic Business Plan to Strategic Mission Plan

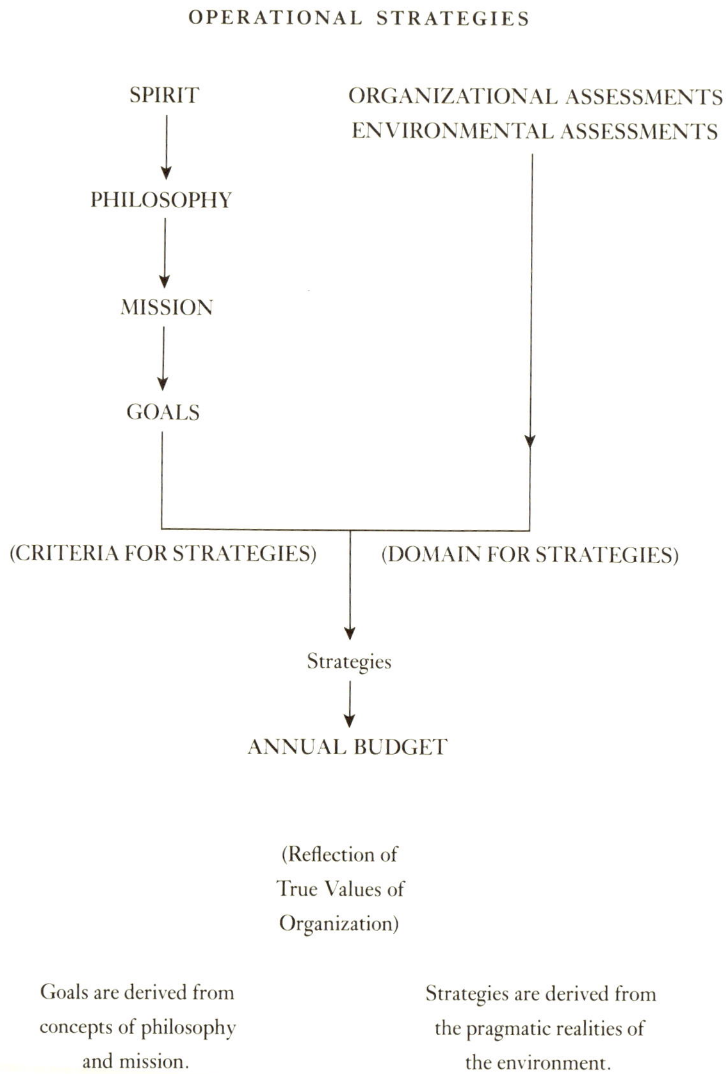

The work of the Daughters of Charity has always focused upon the care of the poor. Perhaps the best-known service at Mary's Help Hospital, on Guerrero Street in San Francisco, was its Clinic, which provided free or low-cost medical and hospital care. Over the years the Clinic maintained its standing as the most highly utilized free clinic in Northern California. The service was continued in Daly City and in satellite Clinics in neighboring communities.

By the 1980s, the Great Society programs—Medicare and MediCal—created a need to find new ways of serving the medically indigent. The Clinic services were revamped to meet current social and health-care needs. For example, in January 1983, the hospital's Clinic organization and name was changed. Individuals and families who for economic reasons do not have access to medical care will continue to have their health-care needs met through what is now called the Family Health Care Service. The hospital has contracted with the Family Medical Group to continue providing medical services to former Clinic members on a free and partial payment basis. In addition, the new program is designed to lower the cost of care and to serve more patients with increased emphasis on primary care and prevention. New satellite physician offices cover a larger geographic area and provide a broader range of services. Bilingual physicians, nurses and clerical personnel are available to assist patients with communication difficulties.

The private, free-standing Family Medical Group provides health care coverage to all financial classes of patients, including those with Medicare, MediCal, prepaid and other private insurance. This facet of the new program creates a more equitable approach to providing health-care for the medically indigent. In the past, these individuals usually received care in separate facilities and within programs that were segregated from the mainstream health-care delivery system. Family Health Care patients, however, receive their care alongside all other types of patients, and there is no discrimination regarding the ability to pay or the type of insurance coverage. Most important, all family members can continue to obtain care from private physicians of their choice as their eligibility for other insurance changes.

In February 1980, we established our Home Health Care Program. This service provides patients with continuing care after they are discharged from the hospital. It assists patients of all ages—from the very young to the elderly. The effects of recuperating in the home are twofold. First, home health care is an alternative to extended hospitalization and, therefore, holds the line on health-care costs while providing comprehensive and quality care. Second, the patient has the advantage of recovering from an illness in the comfort of a familiar environment. The families of patients are also provided with professional and emotional support and assistance.

Although the present structure and operating system of the Home Health Care Department is new, the concept of caring for the ill in their homes is a familiar one to us. The Daughters of Charity have always provided services for the sick outside the walls of the hospital. This service relates in fact to the original charge of St. Vincent de Paul that the Daughters of Charity care for the sick wherever they could be found. This was the first work of the Community.

Today we have one of the best hospital-based home health-care programs in the Bay Area. During the first ten months of the program's existence, our nurses, aides, therapists, and other members of the home care team made 5,500 visits to about 400 patients.

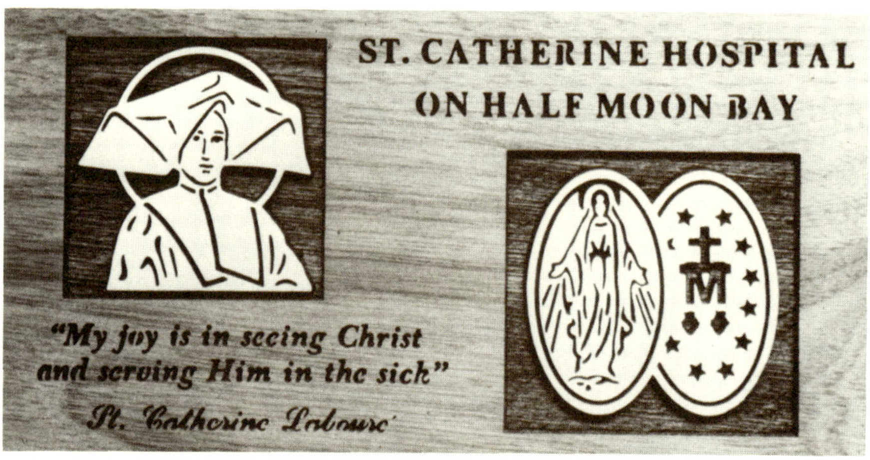
ST. CATHERINE HOSPITAL
ON HALF MOON BAY
"My joy is in seeing Christ
and serving Him in the sick"
St. Catherine Labouré

Reproduction of memento presented on the occasion of the Dedication of St. Catherine Hospital On Half Moon Bay.

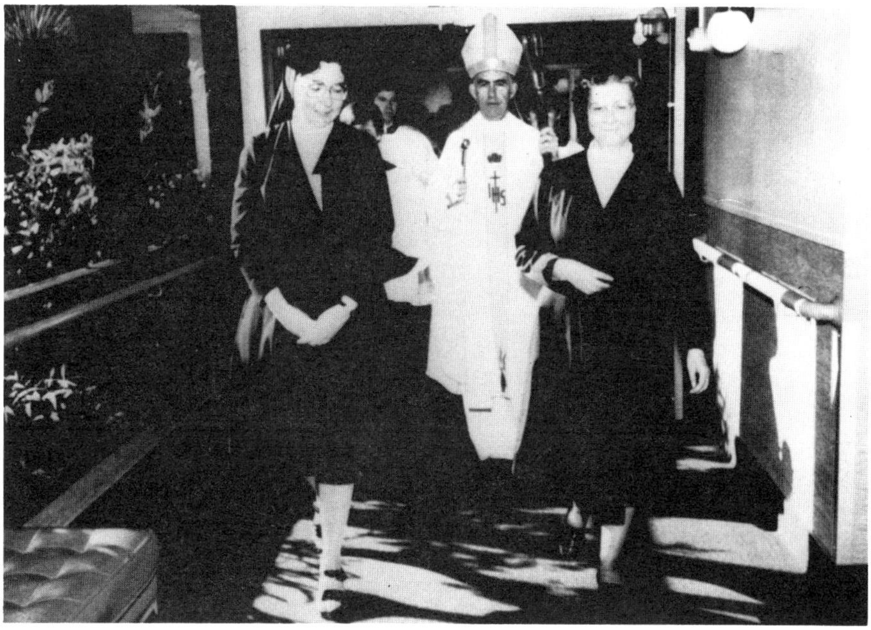

Sister Elizabeth Joseph Keaveney, Archbishop John R. Quinn, and Sister Marie Clare Baldus at the dedication of St. Catherine Hospital On Half Moon Bay, March 5, 1981.

On March 28, 1980, Sister Florence, Chairman of the Board of Directors, Victor Cox, Half Moon Bay Community Board President, and Mayor Albert Adreveno of Half Moon Bay signed the acquisition agreement for the Daughters of Charity to operate the Half Moon Bay Community Hospital. The agreement to sponsor and operate this facility had been made at the request of the Coastside community. The 112-bed facility, which is licensed for 81 skilled nursing beds, 18 women's alcoholic rehabilitation beds, and 13 acute care beds, extends the health-care service area of the Daughters of Charity to Half Moon Bay and the surrounding communities.

On March 5, 1981, the hospital was dedicated by Archbishop John R. Quinn and renamed St. Catherine Hospital On Half Moon Bay. The name honors St. Catherine Labouré, a Daughter of Charity who dedicated her life to caring for the sick and poor. John H. Camaioni, former Associate Administrator at Mary's Help Hospital, has been at St. Catherine Hospital since 1980 and is now Executive Vice-president, Administrator, and Chief Operating Officer.

The Harney Oncology Clinics were the gift of Pauline E. and Charles L. Harney. The center opened on May 11, 1981. A comprehensive program for the care and treatment of cancer patients is provided under the direction of Dr. Barry Chauser.

The Pauline E. and Charles L. Harney Oncology Clinics are structured to meet the complete medical, psychosocial and spiritual needs of patients and their families. Because cancer patients have special needs related to every aspect of their life—from work and family relations to diet and transportation—several hospital departments work together to provide a range of integrated services.

In addition to the three primary modalities of cancer therapy—surgery, chemotherapy and radiation therapy—the program provides counseling, diet planning, support group classes and other services as needed. Physicians and nurses work closely with Social Services and Pastoral Care personnel to help patients and families cope with major decisions and lifestyle changes.

The hospital also provides cancer patients with inpatient care. The individualized style of treatment we provide maximizes continuity of care during the often complex treatment regimens prescribed for patients.

The Radiation Oncology Center, which provides services on both an inpatient and outpatient basis, reinforces the hospital's role as a major center for cancer care in the Bay Area.

An important and progressive component of the oncology services is the hospice program, which provides home care for terminally ill patients. The program is devoted to meeting the needs and wishes of individual patients as comprehensively as possible. Hospice nurses make regularly scheduled home visits to care for the patient and to instruct family members on patient care. Symptoms and pain are controlled without sacrificing the patient's alertness, permitting the enjoyment of family and familiar surroundings as much as is medically feasible.

The search to find a cure for heart disorders is as old as history. The heart has always been regarded as "the seat of the soul and the site of life." For centuries physicians and scientists have devoted their efforts and resources to seeking a solution to heart ailments. The diagnosis and treatment of heart disease made rapid advances following the technological explosion of the 1970s. New knowledge and methodology brought the dream of finding a cure for heart disease a little closer to reality.

We have made a multi-million-dollar investment in cardiovascular facilities to ensure a level of care consistent with the latest technology. A large part of this investment is due to the generosity of the Doelgers, Henry and Thelma. Henry Doelger was the developer of Daly City's Westlake District. The couple provided funds for the Henry Doelger Heart Center and, in addition to the center, the hospital receives an annual disbursement from the Henry Doelger Charitable Trust.

The Henry Doelger Heart Center is a showcase of high technology, with a full range of cardiovascular services, including diagnostic and intervention cardiac catheterization laboratories, physiological testing, coronary care, cardiovascular operating suites, cardiovascular surgical intensive care, and a cardiac rehabilitation program. Cardiovascular surgical procedures performed regularly are coronary bypass surgery, replacement of heart valves, repair of congenital cardiac abnormalities, repair of major blood vessels, and pacemaker implantation and replacements.

In 1982, Dr. Richard K. Myler, one of the developers of percutaneous transluminal coronary angioplasty (PTCA), began using this procedure at the hospital. PTCA is an innovative non-surgical procedure that compresses blockages in arteries by inserting and inflating a tiny balloon in the artery. In many cases it can eliminate the need for open heart surgery. By significantly reducing the risks and expense associated with coronary bypass surgery, PTCA is dramatically altering and simplifying the treatment of coronary artery disease.

In September 1983, we opened the San Francisco Heart Institute, which is dedicated to research and education in the field of cardiovascular disease. Research is devoted to the investigation of both invasive and non-invasive procedures, including PTCA, laser technology, ultra-sound and chemical treatment of acute coronary thrombolysis. Dr. Richard K. Myler is currently Director of the Institute; Dr. Simon H. Stertzer is the Director of Medical Research.

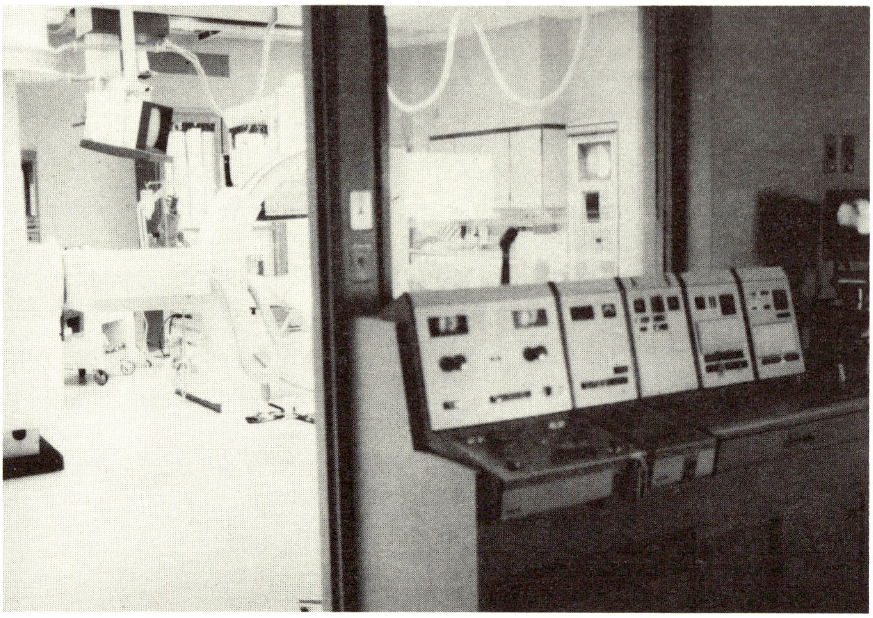

The Henry Doelger Heart Center includes this cardiac catheterization laboratory.

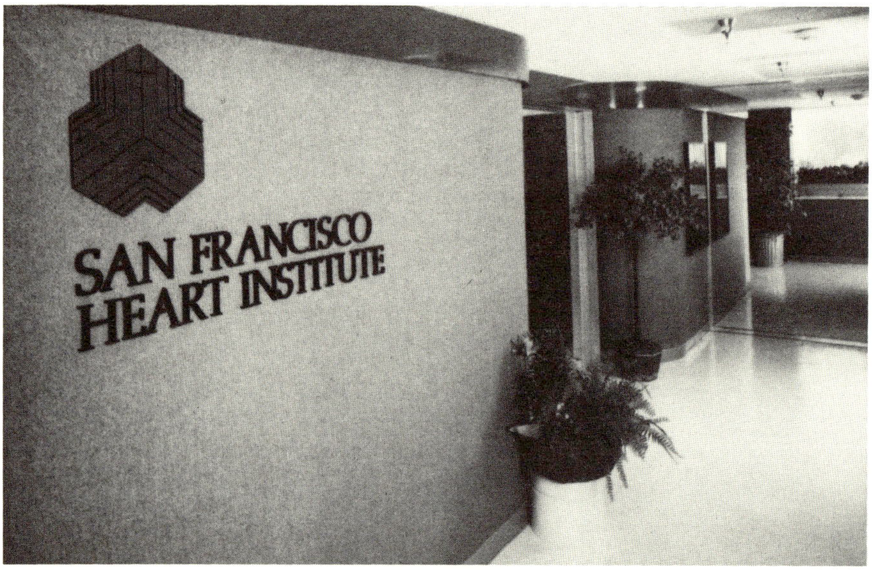

The San Francisco Heart Institute at Seton Medical Center is dedicated to research and education in the field of cardiovascular disease.

The San Francisco Heart Institute supports advanced fellowships in cardiovascular disease, and conducts a broad spectrum of education activities for physicians, nurses, technical staff, and the general public. For example, it sponsors conferences on cardiovascular disease, and physicians from around the world have an opportunity to be in residence at the Institute to learn angioplasty and other current diagnostic and therapeutic procedures.

The range of treatment methods now available to the heart patient extends far beyond what had been the only alternative for centuries—that is, a common weed called purple foxglove (digitalis), which was discovered for its curative properties by William Withering.

The volume of patients seen in the hospital's Emergency Department has tripled during this decade—to about 30,000 patients per year. More important than volume, however, is the fact that we are able to meet the needs of the community by providing accessible hospital services. Volume of patients treated in the Emergency Department also does not speak to the sophistication of the services we provide. Modern equipment and highly trained emergency teams make the Carl Gellert Emergency Center one of the most advanced emergency service systems in Northern California.

In 1981, we became the base station for disasters at the San Francisco Municipal Airport. This contract requires that we serve both San Francisco and San Mateo Counties by coordinating the transfer of disaster victims to receiving hospitals.

New construction in the Emergency Department was completed in 1982. There are presently twelve emergency rooms and seventeen beds. We also contracted with Medevac to provide paramedic services to Daly City, Pacifica, and the Coastside. The paramedic stations are located in the Emergency Departments of Seton Medical Center, Daly City, and St. Catherine Hospital On Half Moon Bay.

On June 25, 1985, we completed the final step in providing services for trauma victims with the opening of the helipad adjacent to the Emergency Department. The helipad permits rapid transfer of trauma victims and other emergency patients to the hospital. It is critical that these patients receive care as rapidly as possible. Time is the single

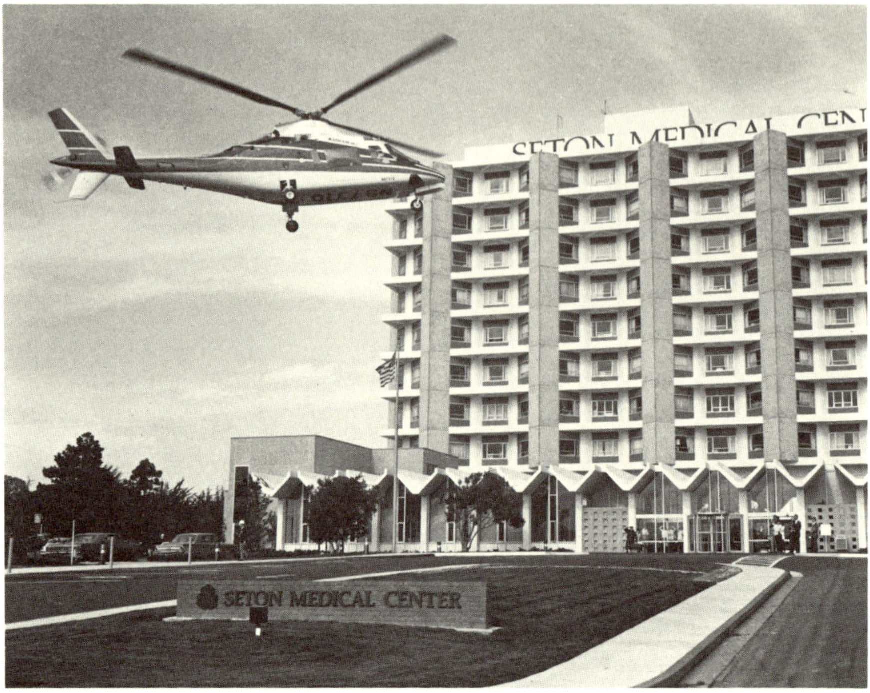

In 1985 a helipad was completed, providing quick access to the hospital during disasters and other emergencies.

most vital element in trauma care. The helipad also provides access to the hospital during disasters when other forms of transportation are not available.

Plans to offer treatment for patients with Hansen's Disease began to take form in 1981. The contract for Mary's Help Hospital to provide this service was signed with the United States Public Health Service on October 28, 1981.

There is no disease with a history as tragic as Hansen's, formerly referred to as leprosy. In the past when the diagnosis was made, the patient became an isolate—physically, socially, emotionally and spiritually. At present, of course, the revolution in therapy offered and the supportive care of these patients has changed dramatically. The range of services now offers patients with Hansen's Disease effective medical treatment and comprehensive support services. The social stigma of the disease has been removed, and the patients usually receive care on an outpatient basis. Hospital care is guaranteed them as well by terms of the contract with the United States Public Health Service.

The total separation of Hansen's Disease victims from society goes back through recorded history, but the present methods of treatment are relatively new. This writer recalls that in the thirties and forties the place of treatment for Hansen's Disease was the Leprosarium in Carville, Louisiana. During my student years affiliating at San Francisco City and County Hospital, now San Francisco General Hospital, a patient diagnosed with Hansen's Disease remained in isolation until several other such patients were seen. They were then transported together to Carville, Louisiana, by a United States Marshal, in an old car purchased exclusively for this purpose.

It is appropriate that patients with Hansen's Disease be treated at a hospital sponsored and operated by the Daughters of Charity. The

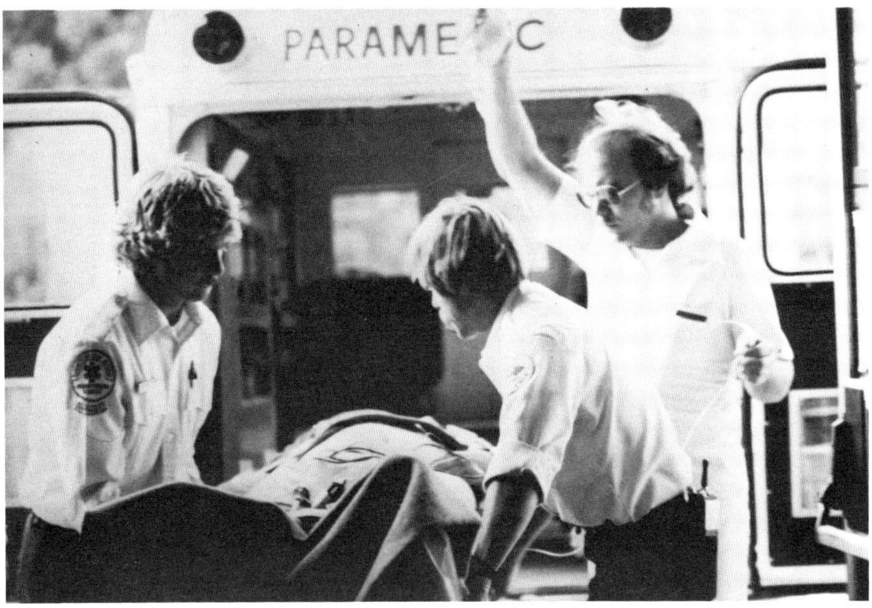

Ambulances arriving at Seton Medical Center.

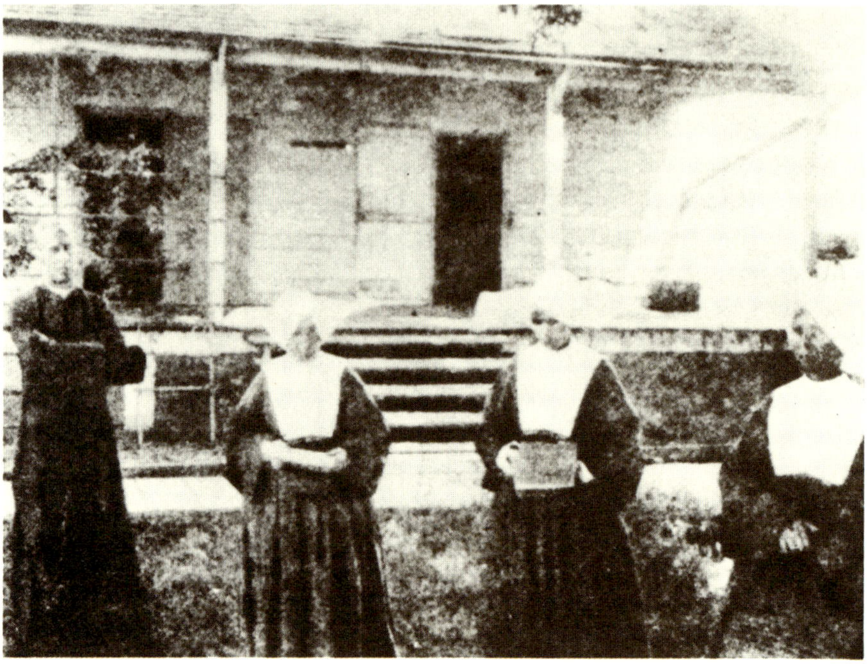

Since 1896 the Daughters of Charity have served Hansen's Disease patients at the United States Government facility in Carville, Louisiana.

Daughters have a long and distinguished history of active care of patients suffering from this disease. In 1896, the Daughters of Charity began serving patients in the Louisiana State Leprosarium in Carville, Louisiana. This institution was acquired by the United States Public Health Service in 1921, and in 1946 it became the National Hansen's Disease Center. The Daughters of Charity remain there today.

This tradition of service to Hansen's Disease patients was extended in 1981 by the Daughters of Charity. With the closure of the United States Public Health Service Hospital in San Francisco, Mary's Help Hospital and the Daughters of Charity were chosen to work with the Public Health Service in continuing the care of Hansen's Disease patients. The administrative transfer from the United States Public Health Service was completed, and all beneficiaries were notified. Dr. Robert Gelber was named Medical Director of the program. Members of our multi specialty Medical/Dental Staff are available for consultation as dictated by patient care needs. The program is staffed by multilingual office personnel, a physical therapist, a home care nurse, social service workers, laboratory technicians and a research technician. Within the first twelve months of the contract, the program was fully active with all services provided.

Most patients come to the Hansen's Disease Clinic at the hospital for outpatient services. Inpatient care is provided as necessary at Seton Medical Center or St. Catherine Hospital. A research program and in-vivo drug sensitivity studies have been in operation since the transfer of the program from the United States Public Health Service.

The Western Hansen's Disease Institute was organized in September 1983, for the purpose of supporting education and research. Members of the Institute include Hansen's Disease clinicians and researchers from San Diego, Los Angeles, San Francisco, Seattle, and Honolulu. The Institute is currently involved in a major serological diagnostic research testing program that may make early diagnosis of Hansen's Disease possible.

No account of Mary's Help Hospital and Seton Medical Center would be complete without a tribute to the women who have participated in the Guild. The first Ladies Auxiliary was formed in 1913. Mrs. M. A. Tobin was President. In the 1930s, the Guild became the St. Louise de Marillac Guild in honor of the canonization of St. Louise in June 1934. The name was changed again in 1950 to the Mary's Help Hospital Guild, and the first President of the reorganized Guild was Dr. Phillis Bourne. In 1983, with the name change of the hospital, the Guild became the Seton Medical Center Guild.

The contributions of the Guild members are legion and cannot possibly be enumerated in this account. From the years 1913 to the present, the assistance of the Guild members has been solicited for virtually every significant hospital activity. They have contributed remarkably to all events. Their activities range from fund raising to providing scholarships for health-care workers. They have given almost one million dollars to the building fund. The generosity of the Guild members reflects their dedication. They have given the work of their hearts, their heads, and their hands to the Sisters and to the hospital.

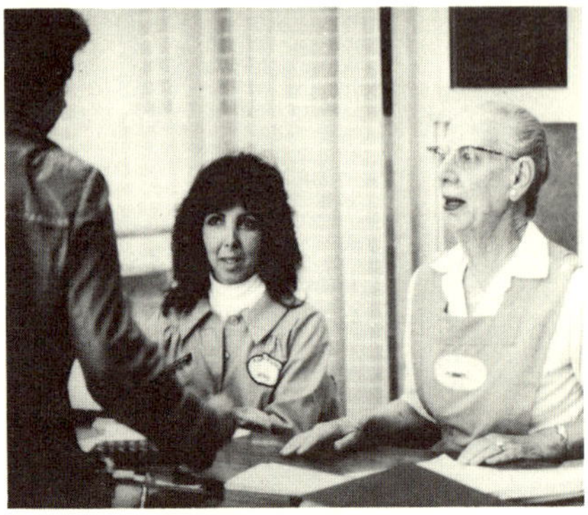
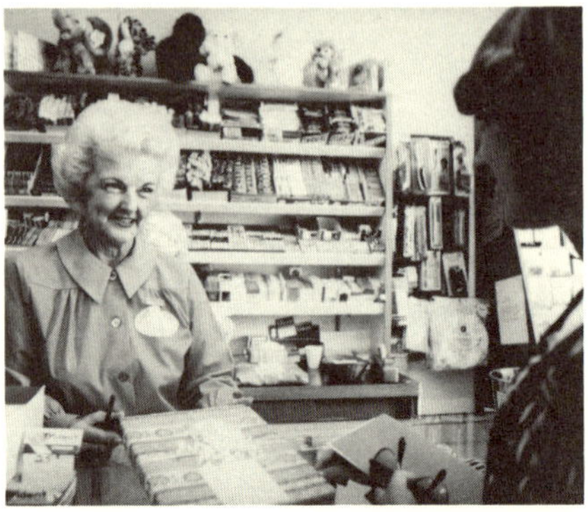
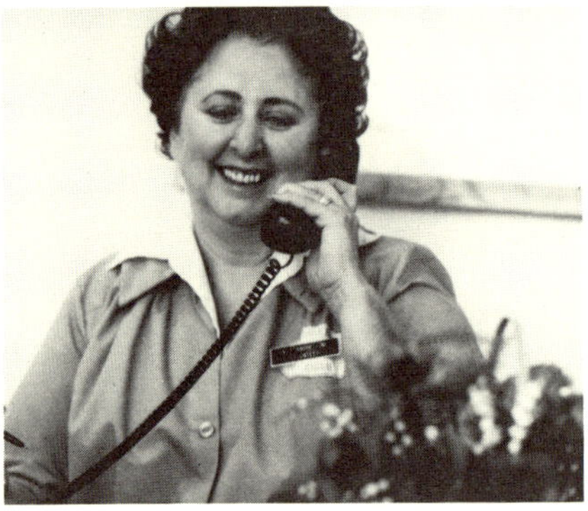
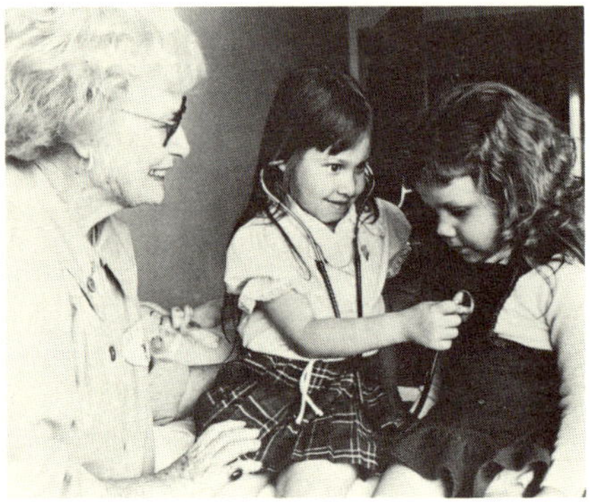

Guild members volunteer throughout the hospital.

On Sunday, April 17, 1983, Mary's Help Hospital was renamed Seton Medical Center. A fifty-five-million dollar building and renovation project, which had started in 1976 in response to rising demands for health care in our service area, was complete. The new facility was dedicated by Archbishop John R. Quinn.

The extensive construction and renovation nearly doubled the square footage of the 1965 structure to one-half-million square feet. The construction provided expanded facilities for the delivery of services in Cardiology, Oncology, Critical Care and Outpatient services. No inpatient beds were added as part of the construction program; therefore, Seton Medical Center remains licensed for 350 beds. The additional facilities enable us to respond fully to community health-care needs ranging from outpatient diagnostic services to open heart surgery. The new facilities and services also definitely established Seton Medical Center as a tertiary health-care facility.

The combined efforts of many diligent workers had brought the project to completion. However, gifts from major donors were the essential component in bringing the dream to fruition. Special facilities made possible by the generous gifts from our benefactors were blessed by Archbishop Quinn at the dedication ceremony. The ceremonies also recognized and honored the donor families. Father John Danagher, C.M., Provincial Director of the Daughters of Charity, offered Mass in the hospital chapel, followed by a reception and the blessing of the special facilities. The ceremonies for donor families were held in the areas made possible by their generosity:

THE HENRY DOELGER HEART CENTER
THE CARL GELLERT EMERGENCY CENTER
THE FRED GELLERT SR. SURGERY CENTER
THE PAULINE E. AND CHARLES L. HARNEY ONCOLOGY CLINICS

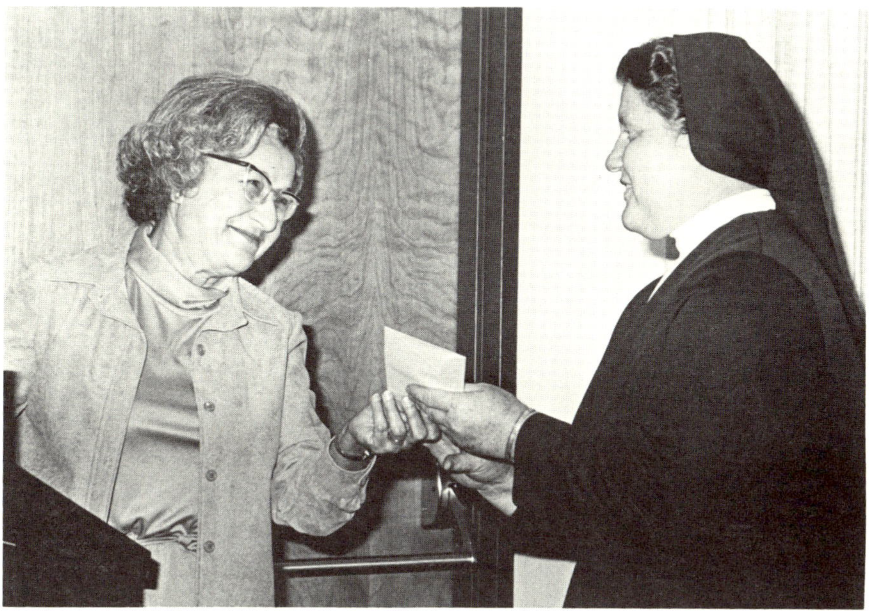

Mrs. Sarah Kelechava, President of Mary's Help Hospital Guild, presents the pledge for the year to Sister Marilynn Emminger, Associate Administrator, Mary's Help Hospital.

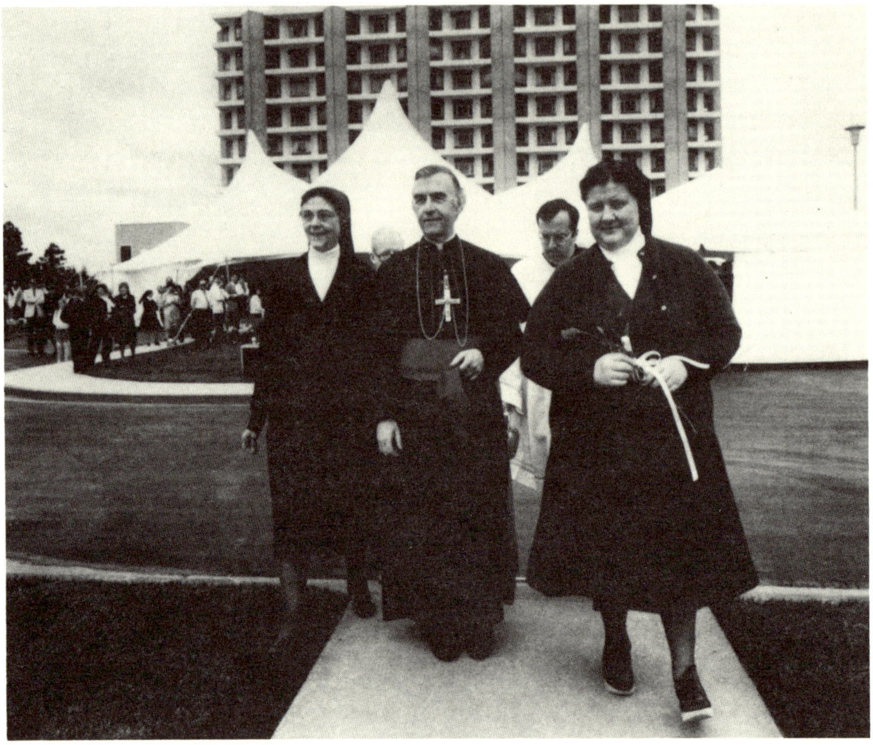

Dedication of Seton Medical Center on Sunday, April 17, 1983. Sister Teresa Piro, Visitatrix; Reverend John Danagher, C.M., Provincial Director of the Daughters of Charity; Archbishop John R. Quinn; Reverend Robert McElroy, Secretary to the Archbishop; and Sister Marilynn Emminger, Health Councillor, Province of the West.

In each location, Archbishop Quinn blessed the dedicatory plaque and the facility. Sister Florence thanked the family members present, and Sister Teresa presented each with a memorial certificate.

The formal dedication ceremony concluded with the blessing of the tree and plaque at the front entrance, which commemorates the living mission of the Daughters of Charity of St. Vincent de Paul. This plaque represents a tribute to the work of the Daughters from November 29, 1633 in Paris to April 17, 1983 in Daly City. The blessing of the tree and the plaque was followed by a reception, an open house and tours for the public. The event concluded that evening with a party in the dedication tent for all the staff who had worked on this successful project.

Simply reading the dedication program does not capture the excitement of the day. There was an element of magic in the ceremony. The balloons, the bands, the banners, the thousands of guests, and the dedication and blessing of the magnificent new structure all represented the culmination of a dream.

Seton Medical Center

Dedication

Sunday, April 17, 1983

San Francisco Boys' Chorus
William Ballard, Music Director

WELCOME
William E. McDonnell, Master of Ceremonies
Vice President
Community Advisory Board

INVOCATION
Very Reverend John J. Danagher, C.M.
Provincial Director of the Daughters of Charity

ADDRESS
The Honorable Louis J. Papan
Assemblyman, 19th District

PLANTING OF THE LIVING MISSION TREE
Rex G. Chase
President & Chief Executive Officer
Seton Medical Center

Edward J. Nino, M.D.
President, Medical/Dental Staff
Seton Medical Center

UNVEILING OF THE STATUE OF ST. ELIZABETH ANN SETON
Sister Teresa Piro, D.C.
Visitatrix, Province of the West

Sister Marilynn Emminger, D.C.
Health Councillor, Province of the West

BLESSING OF SETON MEDICAL CENTER
Most Reverend John R. Quinn, D.D.
Archbishop of San Francisco

Reverend Robert W. McElroy
Secretary to the Archbishop

ADDRESS
The Honorable Jane Powell
Mayor of Daly City

RIBBON CUTTING
Sister Florence Urbine, D.C.
Chairman of the Board
Seton Medical Center

Capuchino High School Marching Band
David Martin, Director

RECEPTION

TOURS

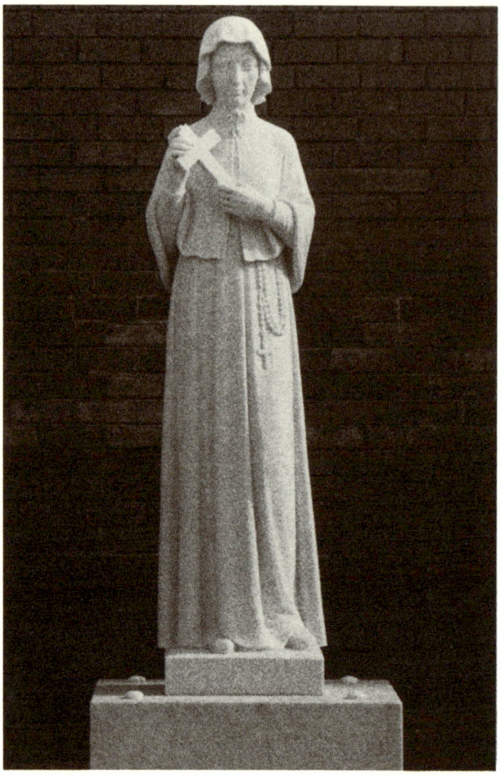

ST. ELIZABETH ANN SETON
This Carrara marble statue faces Seton Medical Center.

Our new name, Seton Medical Center, honors Saint Elizabeth Ann Seton, foundress of the Daughters of Charity in the United States. As part of the dedication ceremony, a statue of Saint Elizabeth Seton, carved in Italy of Carrara marble, was unveiled and dedicated by Archbishop Quinn. It now stands opposite the front entrance of the hospital.

Nineteen hundred eighty-three was a year of celebration: the name change and dedication of Seton Medical Center, and the three hundred and fiftieth anniversary of the founding of the Daughters of Charity of St. Vincent de Paul.

The motto of the Daughters of Charity is: "The Charity of Christ Urges Us." The Daughters of Charity were founded by St. Vincent de Paul and St. Louise de Marillac in Paris, France, on November 29,

1633. The American branch of the Daughters of Charity, which includes about 1700 Sisters in five Provinces, was established in Emmitsburg, Maryland in 1809 by St. Elizabeth Ann Seton. The Daughters of Charity are at present the largest community of religious women in the Roman Catholic Church. Some 32,946 Daughters in 74 geographic provinces throughout the world celebrated their three hundred and fiftieth anniversary in 1983. They continue to serve the poor, the sick and other needy persons in a spirit of humility, simplicity and charity.

Two hundred Daughters of Charity from the Province of the West participated in the anniversary ceremonies on Saturday, November 26, 1983 at St. Mary's Cathedral in San Francisco. It marked the closing of a year of celebration. Archbishop John R. Quinn was principal celebrant and homilist at the Mass of Thanksgiving. A large number of religious and laity whose lives had been touched by the works of the Daughters of Charity were also present.

Today the Daughters of Charity sponsor three health-care institutions in the Bay Area: Seton Medical Center in Daly City, St. Catherine Hospital On Half Moon Bay, and O'Connor Hospital in San Jose. In San Francisco, they also operate one social agency—Mount St. Joseph/St. Elizabeth—and serve at the Alexis Apartments and in Chinatown. The Alexis Apartments are a tribute to Sister Alexis Kuhn, who taught at St. Patrick's Parish for forty-four years. Daughters of Charity also teach in three San Francisco schools: St. Vincent de Paul and Our Lady of the Visitation grade schools, and Cathedral High School. They also work in refugee resettlement at Catholic Social Services in Santa Clara County.

This has also been a time of distinguished visitors. In July 1984, Mother Lucie Rogé, Superioress General, accompanied by Sister Julia Denton, General Councillor, came from the Motherhouse in Paris to visit the works of the Daughters in this area. This was the third time I was privileged to be at the hospital when the Superioress General visited us. I recall other visits: Mother Marie Antoinette Blanchot in 1950 and Mother Francine Lepicard in June 1958.

On January 11, 1985, the Very Reverend Richard McCullen, C.M.,

Superior General of the Congregation of the Mission and of the Daughters of Charity, and the Reverend William W. Sheldon, C.M., Procurator General to the Holy See for the Vincentian Fathers and the Daughters of Charity, visited Seton. This was the first time that the Superior General of the Congregation of the Mission and of the Daughters of Charity had visited the hospital.

The momentum of change in health care was accelerated in 1985. New ways of delivering patient care and service were designed to respond to the challenge of matching needs to contracting resources. We developed an extended outpatient surgical and short-stay service. Our community and patient education programs were assessed and redesigned to meet the needs of patients who now spend less time in the hospital.

One area of the hospital was set up as guest quarters for families of patients or to be used by a patient before surgery. This extension of our hospital service, actually of our hospitality, is looked upon as an innovation; it is not. The origin of the word "hospital" comes from the Latin word "hospitalis," a guest, or host, reminding us that we are returning to our early practice of offering hospitality to patients and their families.

In August 1985 we received the news of the appointment of Frank C. Hudson as President and Chief Executive Officer of Mission Services Corporation, including Seton Medical Center, St. Catherine Hospital On Half Moon Bay, and all other subsidiaries. At the same time, Sister Elizabeth Joseph Keaveney, received her appointment to the position of Executive Vice-president, Mission Services Corporation, and Administrator and Chief Operating Officer of Seton Medical Center. Sister Elizabeth Joseph came to Seton as Vice-President/Senior Associate Administrator in April of 1984.

The newly formed executive team will provide the leadership to continue and to reinforce the mission of the Daughters of Charity in serving the sick and the needy.

December 12, 1985 marked our twentieth anniversary in Daly City. The celebration began at 11 a.m. with Archbishop John R. Quinn offering the Mass of Thanksgiving in the hospital chapel. The Mass was televised throughout the hospital, permitting patients, families, personnel and the overflow of guests to participate. A luncheon followed in the Sisters' residence. Sister Florence Urbine, D.C., Chairman of the Board of Directors, and Frank C. Hudson, President and Chief Executive Officer, welcomed the Archbishop and the honored guests. Jane Powell, former Mayor and current Councilwoman of Daly City, presented Sister Florence with a proclamation from the City of Daly City. Sister Teresa Piro, Visitatrix, Province of the West, presented Archbishop Quinn with a scroll commemorating the eighteenth anniversary of his consecration as a bishop. Sister Teresa's comments as she made the presentation included the recognition that December 12, 1985 was indeed a memorable day marking not just one, but two anniversaries.

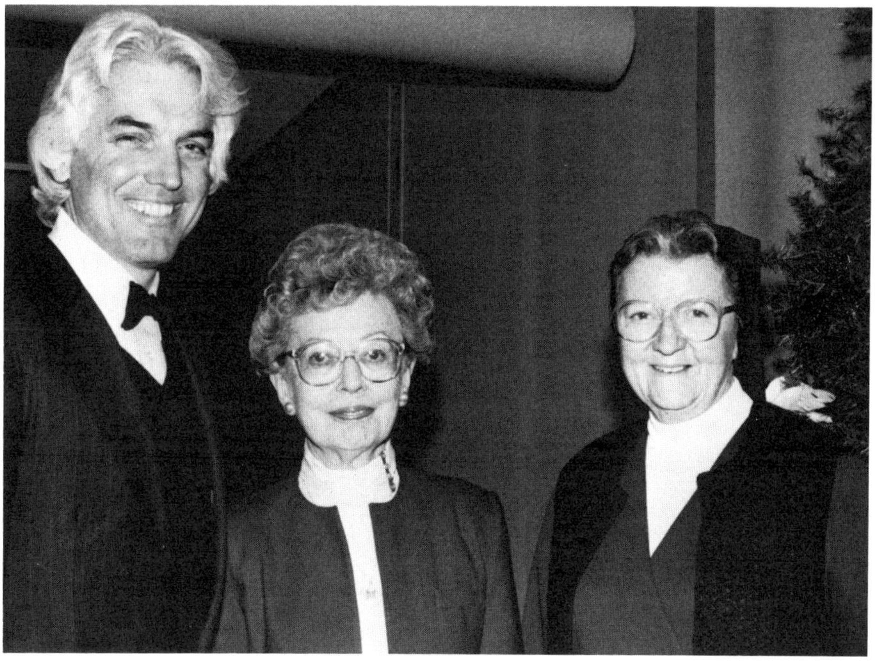

Celebrating the Seton Medical Center's twentieth anniversary in Daly City on December 12,1985: Frank C. Hudson, President and Chief Executive Officer; Marie Mahoney, Assistant to the President; and Sister Florence Urbine, Chairman of the Board of Directors.

Most Reverend John R. Quinn
Archbishop of San Francisco ~

We are privileged to have you with us today to offer the Mass of thanksgiving for our twenty years of service in Daly City ~

We shall continue to strive, at this time of challenge to Catholic health care facilities, to maintain the integration of our core values with our care and cost values. This permits us to provide patient care based on the Philosophy Statement of the Health Care Apostolate of the Daughters of Charity, Province of the West ~

> "We are committed to the ideal that a health care service should contribute to the physical, psychological, social, emotional and spiritual well-being of those served."
>
> "We believe we have the obligation to require an accountability for performance, for adherence to professional and institutional standards, and for adherence to the Ethical and Religious Directives for Catholic Health Facilities as promulgated by the National Conference of Catholic Bishops."

We are grateful to you, Archbishop Quinn, for your support of Seton Medical Center. May you continue to be a visible episcopal presence providing leadership in this time of critical decisions ~

We pray that God will continue to bless you, and most particularly on the eighteenth anniversary of your consecration as bishop ~

Sister Florence Urbine, D.C.
Chairman, Board of Directors ~

Frank C. Hudson
President and
Chief Executive Officer ~

Scroll presented to Archbishop John R. Quinn by Sister Teresa Piro, Visitatrix, commemorating the eighteenth anniversary of his consecration as Bishop.

At the same time, another luncheon and party for all physicians, visitors and employees was in progress in the hospital dining room. This arrangement made it possible for all to participate in our birthday activities.

The growth and expansion we have experienced is due to the involvement and cooperation of all those touched by the organization. Therefore, it was fitting that our festivities were hospital-wide and provided an opportunity to say "Thank You" to all for their dedication to the Daughters of Charity and Seton Medical Center—the dedication which made our hopes and dreams a reality.

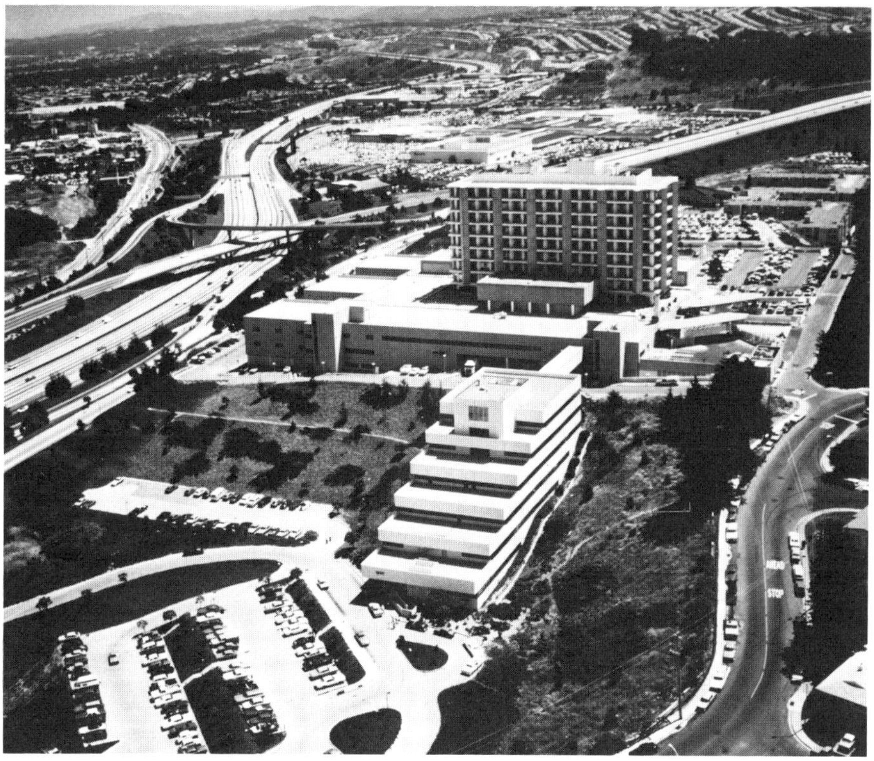

Seton Medical Center overlooks Highway 280 in Northern San Mateo County.

12

The Future

IN CLOSING, I would like to point out that the title, *Reflections on Mary's Help Hospital and Seton Medical Center*, is expressive of the content of this book. Much of the text is my personal recollection of past events, but the title is not rooted in the past. It looks to the future as well. We have experienced the best of both worlds—Mary's Help Hospital and now Seton Medical Center. Mary's Help has bestowed upon Seton an overflow of the spirit. It is a spirit of caring that is uniquely ours. This is our tradition, which is alive and is at present being reinforced and nourished in our patient relations course called "Reflections."

Our history and the traditions of the Daughters of Charity are the major influences upon our present and our future. It is our belief system, our philosophy, and our spirit, expressed as "concern for those who are ill and concern for those who are poor," that energizes us.

This spirit enabled us to grow from a small hospital into a major medical center. The present and future concerns of Seton Medical Center do harken back to our beginnings in San Francisco at the turn of the century. Then, as now, there were regulatory constraints, legal problems, and harsh economic realities. The difficulties of matching resources to needs still challenges us. The solutions then came from the dedication of all involved; the solutions now will come from our commitment to the belief that our role in the future is based on our philosophy.

Embracing the realization of our mission and of our loyalty to the spirit and charism of St. Vincent de Paul, St. Louise de Marillac, and St. Elizabeth Ann Seton, we will respond appropriately to the future challenges—namely, the integration of our core, care, and cost values, and the continuation of our growth as a Catholic health-care facility.

We will continue to strive to reflect our Vincentian Values—the spirit that makes us different!

Appendices

BOARD OF DIRECTORS

Mission Services Corporation / Seton Medical Center

1985

Sister Florence Urbine, D.C., *Chairman*
Sister Rose Collins, D.C., *Vice-Chairman*
Sister Rosalie Larson, D.C., *Secretary and Chief Financial Officer*
Sister Betty Marie Dunkel, D.C.
Sister William Eileen Dunn, D.C.
Sister Marilynn Emminger, D.C.
Sister Mary Genevieve Moonier, D.C.

DAUGHTERS OF CHARITY
AT SETON MEDICAL CENTER
1985

Sister Frances McCarthy, *Sister Servant*
Sister Ursula Chevalier
Sister Alice Mary Devine
Sister Virginia Graham (R.I.P. June 24, 1985)
Sister Aileen Harrington
Sister Elizabeth Joseph Keaveney
Sister Paula Landry
Sister Ann Leitao
Sister Sharon McCarthy
Sister Carmelite O'Connor
Sister Kathleen O'Sullivan
Sister Carmen Ptacnik
Sister Mariana Rabe
Sister Michele Randall
Sister Evelyn Robello
Sister Margaret Salz
Sister Joseph Grace Silvestri
Sister Florence Urbine
Sister Lorraine Valdes

PRESIDENTS OF THE MEDICAL STAFF

MARY'S HELP HOSPITAL
SAN FRANCISCO

A. P. O'Brien, M.D., *First President*
Robert Bilafer, M.D.
Everett Carlson, M.D.
Vincent Derham, M.D.
William Fitzgerald, M.D.
John Golden, M.D.
Alexander Keenan, M.D.
John McGuinness, M.D.
John McQuade, M.D.
Edgar Nolan, M.D.
Theodore Paoli, M.D.
Alfred Reed, M.D.
Francis Rochex, M.D.
Hubert Schwarz, M.D.
Isaac Thorne, M.D.

PRESIDENTS OF THE MEDICAL/DENTAL STAFF

Mary's Help Hospital/Seton Medical Center Daly City

George Torassa, M.D.	1965-1968
Gerald Murphy, M.D.	1968-1969
Werner Disse, M.D.	1969-1971
Samuel McFadden, M.D.	1971-1974
Paul Negulescu, M.D.	1974-1975
Reinold Jones, M.D.	1975-1976
Frank Kmak, M.D.	1976-1977
John Bancroft, M.D.	1977-1978
Robert Brodsky, M.D.	1978-1979
Paul Pitlyk, M.D.	1979-1980
David Young, M.D.	1980-1981
Beth Reimer, M.D.	1981-1982
Edward Nino, M.D.	1982-1983
Paul Fraser, M.D.	1983-1984
Donald Wald, M.D.	1984-1985
Charles Dahlgren, M.D.	1985-

CURRENT MEMBERS OF THE MEDICAL/DENTAL STAFF WHO SERVED AS HOUSE OFFICERS

Mary's Help Hospital/Seton Medical Center

Felix Agcaoili, M.D.
Eugene Baciocco, M.D.
Adolfo Badillo, M.D.
Mario Borja, M.D.
Lucia Cabreros, M.D.
Alberto Consiglieri, M.D.
Rodolfo Duterte, M.D.
Engracia Escobar, M.D.
Alfredo Fernandez, M.D.
Paul Fraser, M.D.
Agaton Gualberto, M.D.
George Keenan, M.D.
Frank Kmak, M.D.
S. C. Liu, M.D.
William Lyden, M.D.
Leonilo Malabed, M.D.
Chris Manitsas, M.D.
Michael McFadden, M.D.
Manuel Morales, M.D.
Mario Mormorunni, M.D.
Gerald Murphy, M.D.
Edgar Nolan, M.D.
Cesar Ortiz, M.D.
Francis Rochex, M.D.
Hubert Schwarz, M.D.
C. Arthur Sciaroni, M.D.
Henry Soldati, M.D.
Elie Tennenbaum, M.D.
Harold Torkelson, M.D.
Reuben Wekselman, M.D.
Norman Wheeler, M.D.
Alan Zacharia, M.D.
John Zucca, M.D.

OFFICERS AND MEMBERS-AT-LARGE
MEDICAL/DENTAL STAFF
Seton Medical Center
1985

Charles Dahlgren, M.D., *President*
Donald Wald, M.D., *Past President*
David Connor, M.D., *President-Elect*
Thomas McGeoy, M.D., *Secretary-Treasurer*
Robert Scribner, M.D., *Member-at-Large*
James Tuzinski, M.D., *Member-at-Large*

DEPARTMENT CHAIRMEN
1985

John Bancroft, M.D., *Department of Orthopedic Surgery*
Thomas Bruce, M.D., *Department of Pathology*
Elias Jacobs, M.D., *Department of Surgery*
Frank Kmak, M.D., *Department of Obstetrics and Gynecology*
Kevin McCarty, M.D., *Department of General and Family Practice*
James Moore, M.D., *Department of Radiology*
Edgar Nolan, M.D., *Department of Medicine*
Marshall Rotterman, M.D., *Department of Anesthesiology*
Robert Saffa, M.D., *Department of Pediatrics*

DIVISION CHIEFS
1985

George Bach-y-Rita, M.D., *Division of Psychiatry*
Bruce Dobbs, D.P.M., *Division of Podiatry*
William Dowling, M.D., *Division of Oncology*
Philip Hertz, M.D., *Division of Nephrology*
Reinold Jones, M.D., *Division of Cardiothoracic Surgery*
Robert Kradjian, M.D., *Division of General Surgery*
Thomas McGeoy, M.D., *Division of Urology*
Sean Moloney, M.D., *Division of Plastic Surgery*
Neil Mulcahy, M.D., *Division of Otolaryngology*
Paul Pitlyk, M.D., *Division of Neurosurgery*
D. Richard Reynolds, M.D., *Division of Ophthalmology*
Richard Robert, D.D.S., *Division of Oral Surgery and Dentistry*
Anthony Russo, M.D., *Division of Pulmonary Medicine*
Colman Ryan, M.D., *Division of Cardiology*
Robert Scribner, M.D., *Division of Vascular Surgery*
Robert Telfer, M.D., *Division of Neurology*
Leo van der Reis, M.D., *Division of Gastroenterology*

COMMUNITY ADVISORY BOARD

Seton Medical Center

June 1985

Mr. William E. McDonnell, *Chairman*
Mr. James C. Wyatt, *Vice-Chairman*
Mr. Edward Barry
Mr. Henry Bostwick, Jr.
Mr. John Brucato
Mr. Patrick Cannon
Mrs. Roy Carter
Mr. Hugh Connolly
Mrs. Marian H. Conser
Mrs. James Cooper
Mr. William G. Crocker
Ms. Margaret M. Cummins
Mrs. Eleanor Davis
Mr. Jack Donnellan
Mr. Henry M. Duque
Mr. William J. Dwyer
Mr. Jose P. Flores
Mr. Elio Fontana
Dr. Floyd Gonella
Mr. Dale A. Hauch
Mr. Jack Hickey
Mrs. Hugo Holmstrom
Mr. Gerald Kelly
Mr. George Kiesel

Mr. Edward M. King
Mr. Louis Cal LaLanne
Mr. Rod MacDonald
Mr. Peter Markovich
Mr. James F. Maxwell
Mr. Dan Modena
Mrs. Theodore Paoli
Mr. Daniel Pommon
Mrs. Jane Powell
Mr. Gilbert Salas
Mr. James Scatena
Mr. John E. Sullivan
Mr. Mel Tafoya
Mr. Michael R. Wyman

HONORARY MEMBERS OF THE COMMUNITY ADVISORY BOARD

Seton Medical Center

Mr. Vincent Cullinan
Mr. James Cummins
Mrs. Curtis Day
Mr. Dennis Jordan
Mr. Francis P. Pacelli
Mr. James Rudden

PRESIDENTS OF THE GUILD

Prior to 1950 Reorganization

Mrs. M. A. Tobin, *First President*
Mrs. Robert Bilafer
Miss Marie Hayden
Mrs. George Littlejohn
Mrs. J. Marinetti
Mrs. William Mullane
Mrs. A. P. O'Brien
Mrs. John O'Toole

PRESIDENTS OF THE GUILD

From 1950 Reorganization to Present

Dr. Phillis Bourne	1950-1952
Julia Golden (Mrs. John)	1952-1953
Loretta O'Grady (Mrs. William)	1953-1954
Blanche Gardner (Mrs. Henry)	1954-1955
Enid Paoli (Mrs. Theodore)	1955-1956
Peggy Gobar (Mrs. Robert)–Resigned, health reasons	1956-1957
Dr. Phillis Bourne filled her unexpired term	
Dr. Phillis Bourne	1957-1958
Marybelle Nolan (Mrs. Edgar)	1958-1959
Helen Sanchez-Corea (Mrs. Antonio)	1959-1961
Elaine Pope (Mrs. Thomas)	1961-1962
Eve Duval (Mrs. Hunter)	1962-1963
Mary Neagle (Mrs. Paul)	1963-1964
Bernadette Price (Mrs. Warren)	1964-1965
Helen Vollert	1965-1966
Sarah Kelechava (Mrs. Frank)	1966-1967
Terry Mortara (Mrs. Fred)	1967-1968
Helen Corbett (Mrs. William)	1968-1969
Eleanor West (Mrs. Clifton)	1969-1970
Kay Glebow (Mrs. Philip)	1970-1971
Evelyn Fitzgerald (Mrs. J. J.)	1971-1972
Millie Dunow (Mrs. Cal)	1972-1973
Mary Short (Mrs. Elwin)	1973-1974
Frances Gaffigan (Mrs. Milton)	1974-1975
Virginia Stanghellini (Mrs. Thomas)	1975-1977
Sarah Kelechava (Mrs. Frank)	1977-1979
Jane Hillsman (Mrs. Carlyle)	1979-1981
Marie Michalske (Mrs. Donald)	1981-1982
Alyce Brachman	1982-1984
Grace Carboni (Mrs. Vincent)	1984-

Bibliography

Bancroft, Hubert Howe: *History of California.* San Francisco: The History Company, 1888.

Bronson, William: *The Earth Shook, The Sky Burned.* Garden City: Doubleday and Company, 1959.

Dirvin, Joseph I., C.M.: *Mrs. Seton, Foundress of the American Daughters of Charity.* New York: Farrar, Strauss & Giroux, 1975.

Hogan and German: *The Great Epidemic.* Boston: Little, Brown and Company, 1961.

MacEachern, Malcolm T.: *Hospital Organization and Management.* Chicago: Physicians' Records, 1951.

Meyers, Sister Bertrande, D.C.: *Then and Now with the Daughters of Charity.* St. Louis: Vincentian Press, 1946.

Ryan, Andrew M., M.D.: "Mary's Help Hospital Over The Years, 1889–1965." May 1965.

Tyler, Sidney: *San Francisco's Great Disaster.* Philadelphia: P. W. Zeigler Co., 1906.

Other Sources

Documents, minutes, and records from the Archives of the Archdiocese of San Francisco, California.

Documents, minutes, and records from the Archives of the Board of the Corporation, Mary's Help Hospital, San Francisco, California.

Documents, minutes, and records from the Archives of the Mary's Help Hospital and Seton Medical Center Board of Directors, Daly City, California.

Records and clippings from the Archives of Seton Provincialate, Los Altos Hills, California.

Education News & Notes from Mary's Help Hospital and Seton Medical Center, Daly City, California.

Records from the Mary's Help Hospital and Seton Medical Center Guild, San Francisco and Daly City, California.

Minutes and records from Mary's Help Hospital and Seton Medical Center Medical/Dental Staff, Daly City, California.

Minutes and records from Mary's Help Hospital Nurses Alumnae Association, San Francisco and Daly City, California.

Daughters of Charity of St. Vincent de Paul

Serving in Health, Education, and Social Ministry

This book has been designed by Marianne Hinckle
and printed by Thomson Lithograph, Inc., on Mohawk Superfine #80 Text.
Text and display type was set by Mackenzie-Harris Corporation
in *Jansen* on the Mergenthaler 202. Editions were bound in Van Heek
Almoline cloth by Cardoza James Binding Co. Production assistance
from Madeleine Corson, Patricia Glover and Adelaida Mejia.
Cover design executed by Madeleine Corson.
Frontispiece illustration by Joseph S. Cleary.

This book was designed
and produced by
Hinckle & Sons
Printing Office

SAN FRANCISCO